CRITICAL PUBLISHING

DEVELOPING YOUR
PROFESSIONAL
IDENTITY

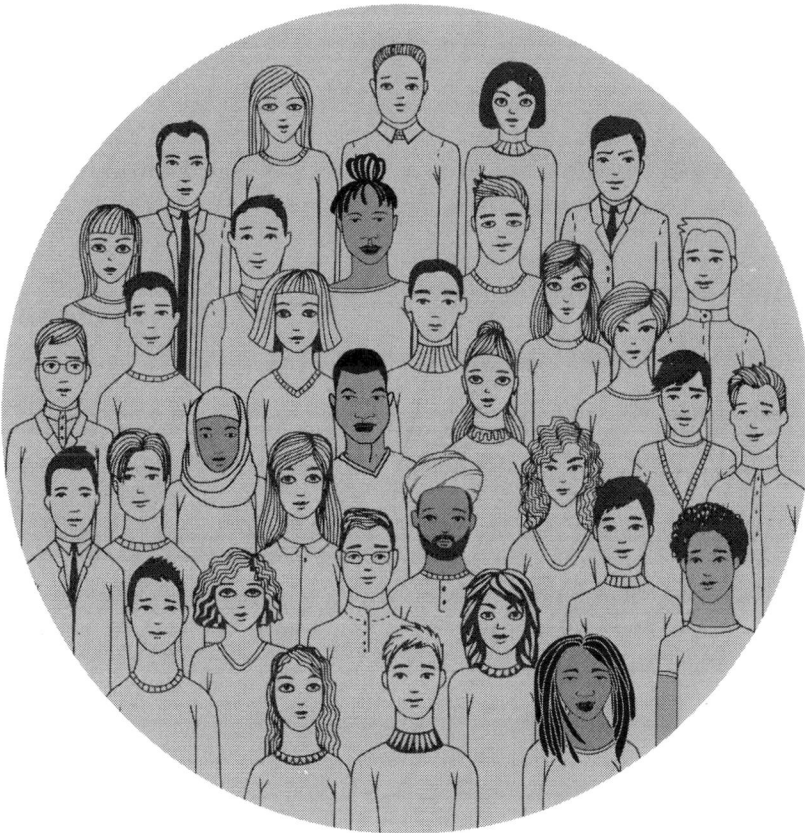

A GUIDE FOR WORKING
WITH CHILDREN AND FAMILIES

Edited by Hazel Richards and Michelle Malomo

First published in 2022 by Critical Publishing Ltd

British Library Cataloguing in Publication Data
A CIP record for this book is available from the British Library

ISBN: 978-1-914171-53-6

This book is also available in the following e-book formats:

EPUB ISBN: 978-1-914171-54-3
Adobe e-book ISBN: 978-1-914171-55-0

Cover design by Out of House Limited
Text design by Greensplash
Project management by Newgen Publishing UK
Printed and bound in Great Britain by 4edge, Essex

Critical Publishing
3 Connaught Road
St Albans
AL3 5RX

www.criticalpublishing.com

Printed on FSC accredited paper

DEVELOPING YOUR
PROFESSIONAL
IDENTITY

A GUIDE FOR WORKING
WITH CHILDREN AND FAMILIES

To order, or for details of our bulk discounts, please go to our website www.criticalpublishing.com or contact our distributor, Ingram Publisher Services (IPS UK), 10 Thornbury Road, Plymouth PL6 7PP, telephone 01752 202301 or email IPSUK.orders@ingramcontent.com.

Contents

Part 3 Succeeding amid work-based learning issues

Part 4   Moving forwards

Dedications

For Shona and all her peers who showed me – and who have kept going through such challenging times.

Hazel

To Mum: your strength despite adversity has inspired me to always keep trying; even when life is tough your influence lives on.

To Anya: your passion for being the best version of you in all things has inspired me to write this book for all those of your generation, hoping that together you can change the world with kindness and compassion.

To Abiodun: who reminds me that all will be well.

Michelle

About the book editors

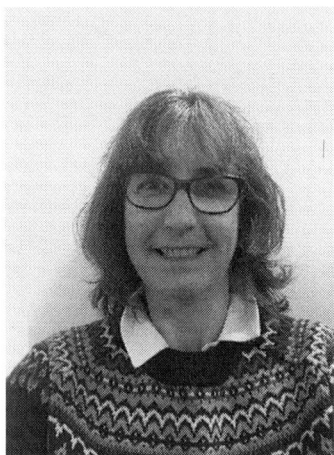

Hazel Richards

Hazel is a registered Speech and Language Therapist and has worked with children with complex needs in mainstream and specialist settings, including CAMHS, for many years. Following her Masters in special and inclusive education, she moved to further education to work with young people with acquired brain injury. Her passion for supporting and developing professional practice led to her doctoral studies, which investigated SENCo identity and influences on practice. She lectured at the University of Worcester in education studies and for the Department of Children and Families before moving to the University of Wolverhampton, where she is a senior lecturer in special educational needs, disability and inclusion studies.

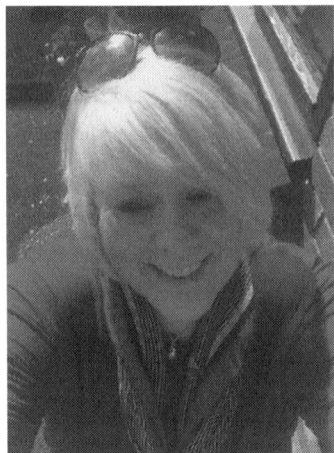

Michelle Malomo

Michelle is currently a senior lecturer and partnership co-ordinator for the FdA in the early years (0–8) at the University of Worcester. Having started work as a nanny and then as a nursery manager, early years practice became a passion. During this time Michelle worked closely with practitioners who wanted to train while on the job and this developed her skills and enthusiasm for work-based learning. Michelle also has a passion for the power and value of play as a therapeutic approach for children and young people's well-being. She has worked within the playwork field and appreciates the value of play for children within their communities. Outside of work Michelle has volunteered as a youth worker.

About the authors

Angela Hodgkins is a senior lecturer at the University of Worcester. Her professional background is in nursery nursing, teaching in FE and HE, and counselling. Angela is a course leader and she teaches a range of subjects, including reflective and professional practice. She is currently studying for a PhD looking at early years practitioners' empathy within their role. Empathy and emotional intelligence are her main research interests. Angela is also a Senior Fellow of the Higher Education Academy.

Emma Laurence is a primary school teacher who is currently studying for a PhD in educational leadership with the University of Worcester. Her research explores how headteachers are supported by their professional networks. She has a BA in early childhood and an MA in education.

Alison Prowle is a senior lecturer in the Department of Children and Families at the University of Worcester. She teaches across a range of programmes, specialising in adverse childhood experiences, human trafficking and forced migration, and strength-based family support. Prior to entering academia, Alison worked extensively in education, community development and social care, most recently holding the position of Head of Preventative Services for Children, Young People and Families for a Welsh local authority.

Erica Strudley-Brown is a Senior Fellow at The University of Worcester and Vice President of Acorns Children's Hospices. Erica has longstanding experience working with children with complex needs as a deputy headteacher and as a headteacher in special schools. In recent years she has worked as a principal lecturer and senior research fellow in higher education. She has published extensively in subjects related to special education, children's palliative care and bereavement. Erica has been made a Fellow of the Royal Society of Arts in recognition of her contribution to working with families facing adversity.

Samantha Sutton-Tsang is course leader for the foundation degree in early years (flexible and distributed learning pathway) at the University of Worcester. She has worked in early years settings as a practitioner, as a primary school teacher and lecturer in further education. Her teaching and research interests include technology-enhanced learning and supporting students with their research in practice. Samantha is a Senior Fellow of the Higher Education Academy.

Rosie Walker is an associate lecturer, having recently retired as a senior lecturer in children and families at the University of Worcester. Professionally, she is a qualified social worker and has worked in a variety of social care roles and managed two large children's centres within the UK. She has written and co-edited several books, including *Mentoring and Coaching in Early Childhood Education*. Her research interests include critical thinking and social justice within higher education. She is a Senior Fellow of the Higher Education Academy.

Acknowledgements

We are indebted to the many people who gave generously of their time and expertise in order to produce this book. First, we would like to acknowledge the contribution of all the authors who delivered timely and well-researched chapters. Their professionalism and willingness to meet deadlines and respond to the comments of the reviewers made editing this book a pleasure.

Particular thanks go to the children, young people, students and colleagues who provided the case studies. As the book is aimed at students and practitioners it seems wholly appropriate that front-line, lived experience and voices are foregrounded and these honest and sometimes raw accounts bring the text to life for us.

We would also like to acknowledge the generosity of www.boingboing.org.uk/ who happily offer their resilience frameworks for free (see Figure 4.2, Chapter 4).

Our thanks also go to our respective institutions, the Department of Children and Families at the University of Worcester and the Department for Special Educational Needs and Disability Studies at the University of Wolverhampton, both of whom have been highly supportive and understanding throughout the process.

We would also like to thank our respective families, who have provided much needed moral support and understanding, and who are, in many ways, the inspiration for the book.

Finally, we would like to thank Julia Morris at Critical Publishing who has provided unfailingly wise and responsive guidance.

Introduction

This book arose from our awareness as experienced practitioners and tutors supporting students to develop the skills and resilience needed in practice. We are passionate about equipping students to be effective and resilient, a goal brought into sharp focus by the pandemic. Covid-19 required our students to work as key workers and to transition very suddenly into positions of responsibility. They had to meet increasingly demanding scenarios while also juggling the challenges inherent in being new practitioners and tests the pandemic created in their own personal lives.

The catalyst for the book was what we were experiencing in student tutorials and the stories from practice we were hearing. This identified to us an increased need to 'care for the carers'. Indeed, the realities of the pandemic meant that workplace programmes of support for transitioning into the early stages of qualified practice or new roles were, in many cases, reduced or non-existent – a situation that happened alongside reduced peer contact and outlets for social support. We know that children and family work can transform outcomes and so the lives of individuals. We also know that the practitioners involved in such work are often highly motivated and conscientious and that work with children and their families can be taxing and, at times, highly emotional.

The aim of this book is therefore to support students and newly qualified practitioners to develop the attributes and skills that will support their well-being and professional practice. The book also explores areas to consider as you develop your professional identity. It does not, however, give you formulas or facile answers. Rather, it invites you to explore your own responses to the ideas it contains so that you develop your own personal toolkit. This means you might favour one tool over another, and that your priorities or need for different tools will change, depending on the situation and your experience. We ourselves have very different backgrounds and experience. For example, Hazel is a Speech and Language Therapist used to a measure of formal reflection in the form of clinical supervision, whereas Michelle was an Early Years Manager for whom this is a newer concept. Certainly, one thing the pandemic has taught us is that everyone has their own story or experiences and there is great diversity with the roles each of you hold in supporting children and families.

But there is this common value which is the work we do – and our motivation and passion to see the very best outcomes for the children and families that you work with. We have therefore called on students and recently qualified practitioners to contribute to the book, and their stories, for us, are what bring it to life. As Berardi (2017, p 203) said, '*The autonomy of knowledge is not a philosophical issue. It is a social issue as it is based on the concrete potency of concrete social actors*'. '*Developing your professional identity: a guide for working with children and families*' therefore recognises that you, as social actors, have the power to support and strengthen your agency and that such strength enables your practice to have a transformative effect on the lives of the children and families that you work with. However, the need for self-care is increasingly recognised since it is important that you are able to care for others without losing yourself, meaning constant and persistent reflection are encouraged throughout the book.

All chapters follow a similar format with each taking a solutions-focused approach to a different aspect of identity or practice. Beginning with aims and an introduction to the topic, every chapter explores theory and contemporary issues. Points to reflect on in the form of time to consider and critical questions are used at key points throughout each chapter. The purpose of these is to either progress your knowledge of yourself and your setting (time to consider) or interrogate and develop your perspectives (critical questions). These may take some time to solve and you may find that you have to carry these with you and ponder on them. Case studies are also used in most chapters to bring theory to life. Reading stories of others can touch our own experience of practice as well as provide examples of real-life application of the theories and research findings presented. Finally, all chapters end with a summary of the key points and signposts to further reading or resources that will enable you to build up your bank of knowledge and solutions.

The book is divided into four sections. The first section contains two chapters that support you to recognise the power of work-based learning. Chapter 1 explores the multifaceted nature of our identities and how these interact to inform the perspectives and actions of practitioners. The chapter goes on to explore factors that may constrain or enable the power you have to act and speak out in your work to support and better outcomes for children and families. Chapter 2 recognises that work with children and their families involves diverse, novel and sometimes challenging situations where there is no 'off the shelf' solution. It explores reflection as a means to critically and objectively consider the multiple perspectives and issues present in situations in order to identify possible responses and courses of action. The chapter identifies that reflection is a very personal process, so different models and strategies are explored, and it is suggested that applying reflection, not just to your practice but also to learn about yourself, your strengths and challenges, and when and how you need to be kind to yourself as a practitioner is a vital part of developing your professional identity.

This leads us in to the second section of the book, which considers the importance of caring for yourself as a work-based learner. Central to this is the importance of self-care in supporting your well-being, which is explored in Chapter 3. The chapter identifies key areas to consider and signposts you to a range of solutions and strategies to choose from. Chapter 4 aims to progress your understanding of resilience, and how resilience can help you navigate the challenges and adversities that come your way. It proposes that resilience can be developed within individuals by progressing an understanding of self and by certain strategies and tools. Chapter 5 proposes that empathy is an essential element of working with children and families, since it makes us compassionate and helps us to build the close relationships which are so important in our professions. The chapter also explores what the impact of the sometimes highly emotional work involved with child and family support work might be on the practitioner and looks at ways of minimising burnout in practice.

The third section of the book addresses issues you may encounter in the course of your work-based learning. Chapter 6, entitled '*Finding your place in safeguarding practice*', recognises that while safeguarding and keeping safe is a central aspect of child and family support work, these can feel like a risky element of our practice. The chapter acknowledges that we may need to build courage and that emotions may be stirred, but in keeping with the solutions-focused tenor of the book, the chapter also aims to equip students to take advantage of opportunities to learn through reflective practice so that they can make a critical contribution to inter-agency practice. Chapter 7 then presents children's understanding of adverse life events and their responses to these events. Throughout the chapter, the voices of real children are used to provide a powerful insight into their lived experience and so enhance our understandings. The chapter also acknowledges that because we are all different, the ways in which we react in the face of such adversity, and the coping strategies which we adopt as practitioners will be unique to each of us. Chapter 8 goes on to explore the important contribution healthy workplace relationships make since where positive relationships exist, practitioners will be supported, and challenged, to progress their skills and horizons. It suggests that communication and a growth mindset are key to the effective teamwork essential to proficient child and family work. The last chapter of Part 3, Chapter 9, considers how coaching and mentoring can develop your professional identity and support your work, how this might best work for you, and how you can influence and make the best use of what is offered at your setting.

The last section of the book is concerned with your step forwards into qualified practice. You do not enter your post qualification role as a fully completed practitioner. Chapter 10 therefore explores stages involved in transitioning to independent practice, along with support and strategies that can help you successfully progress. Certainly, your identity is likely to change significantly during this period, as you evolve from student to novice to independent practitioner.

This continued development and learning is something we definitely recognise and value both as practitioners and as educators. While we have years of experience between us, we ourselves can identify how much our own identities, practice and solutions have developed throughout the course of, and as a result of creating this book. We are also thrilled the case study contributors, who were each given the context of the chapter they were writing for, benefited from the process. Comments such as '*I kind of enjoyed writing it and I am okay with my real name being used in the case study as it makes me feel quite important!*' (Hamida, Chapter 1); '*I really enjoyed reading the section of the chapter and felt I could really relate to what was said*' (Sophie, Chapter 10); and '*Oh my gosh I'm so pleased that you liked it! Was quite a lovely experience just taking a second to reflect on everything that's happened. Thank you so much again, and super excited to eventually read the final chapter and the book*' (Laura, Chapter 10) affirmed to us the purpose and place this book has.

We hope you enjoy this book, and that you learn and can apply the content as much as we have. Indeed, our hope is that as you read the book your professional identity development will progress to a new and exciting place, and that the learning and strategies you take from it will empower you to stand within and progress practice in the sector. We also hope the book will be something that you dip into as you transition into the practitioners of the future and progress your career. We wish you well and we are proud of each and every one of you.

Hazel and Michelle

Reference

Berardi, F (2017) *Futurability: The Age of Impotence and the Horizon of Possibility.* London: Verso.

Part 1 Recognising the power of work-based learning

1 Developing your identity, agency and voice

HAZEL RICHARDS

Chapter objectives ◎

This chapter considers the place of identity, agency and voice in your practice. The chapter:

- uses theory to build your understanding of these concepts;
- poses critical questions to enable you to reflect on your own identity, agency and voice;
- considers emerging research; and
- proposes how you can empower your identity, agency and voice.

Time to consider ☁

» Who are you as a practitioner and what do you bring?

» What do you already know about identity, agency and voice?

Introduction

Children and family support workers are often driven by altruism and moral capital since they are empowered to actions that will create change and betterment. Politics, values and ethics merge to create practitioners who believe in the worth of such work. This chapter investigates theory surrounding the concepts of identity, agency and voice which are central to this, since such knowledge can help you to shape your responses, empower your practice and maintain your sense of social agency.

Theory and literature

Identity

Identity, as a person's source of meaning and motive, is central in informing how individual practitioners carry out their job roles and responsibilities. Identity has been defined in different ways – as a stable, unchanging essence (Cooley, 1902) and also as an evolving state (Mead, 1934; Giddens, 1991). Theorists have grappled to describe what contributes to identity. Korsgaard (2009) suggests values underpin identity so orienting life around personally meaningful projects is important. Mollenhauer (2014) uses the German word *bildung* (which describes the process of self-cultivation and maturation) to suggest that identity emerges from the harmonisation of the mind and heart. This can be problematical since there may be a mismatch between our desires and the actualisation of these. For that reason, Ball (1972) separates a core presentation of self that is fundamental to how a person thinks from another, malleable, identity that adapts according to the context or situation. Erikson (1959) also recognised this difference, suggesting that we all have a real (forever revised and what we are able to attain within social reality) and ideal identity ('*a set of to-be-strived-for but forever-not-quite-attainable ideal goals for the self*', p 140).

Jenkins (2004) therefore suggests humans can be best understood in terms of their personal, professional and collective selves, and that these interact and inform the philosophies and belief systems that drive our actions. Indeed, your personal identity is central to your performance of professional roles since who you are and what you bring influences the way you construe and carry out your work. Professional identity is concerned with role identity, which is connected with subject and job knowledge, as well as with professional ideals, goals and values. External conditions (professional knowledge, context of setting and wider educational contexts) contribute to the formation of professional identity through '*socialisation and absorbing values*' (Phillips and Dalgarno, 2017, p 2). An interrelationship between personal and professional identities therefore exists, with one informing the other. Significantly, strong professional identity constructions, which influence high levels of professional practice, are created when mismatches between who practitioners are as people, and what they do in practice, are worked through (Callero, 1985).

'*Biographicity*' is a term denoting individual responses to social conditions (Illeris, 2014, p 152). Collective identity is therefore also important since viewpoints created by individual experience are influenced by societal conditions and by environments. This means the beliefs and attitudes you hold, can align with, or be challenged and modified by factors in the contexts and settings you work in. Furthermore, commitment (to a team or a setting) is affected by an individual's sense of being included and belonging, with identity having a key influence on the sustained commitment and motivation of educational professionals (Jo, 2014; Vähäsantanen, 2015). In contrast, feeling peripheral affects self-esteem, motivation and collaboration, which can impact on the agency of practitioners (Isaksson and Lindqvist, 2015).

Time to consider

» How is your professional identity developing? How would you like it to develop further?

» Identify a time when your values conflicted with a task undertaken as part of your role? What helped you address and overcome this?

» When have you experienced the strongest sense of belonging at work and what contributed to this?

Agency

Agency refers to the thoughts and actions taken by persons that express their individual power (Bourdieu, 2002). Taylor (1985) describes a human agent as one who has some understanding of self. Professional agency represents the idea that professionals have the power to take stances, make decisions and influence matters. However, agency is not '*solely lodged in the body of an individual agent*' (Van de Putte et al, 2017, p 885), and constraints, such as stress and workload can restrict it. In practice, we are part of an '*intra-active entanglement of multiple agencies*' (Van de Putte et al, 2017, p 885), with agency being linked to status in multidisciplinary working (Meyer and Lees, 2013). However, defining agency is difficult. Some suggest professional agency is '*practiced*' by being able to influence one's work and professional identity (Taylor, 1985). Others define agency as a '*capability*' (Pyhältö et al, 2015). An alternative definition is offered by Biesta et al (2016, p 626), who describe it as an '*actor–situation transaction*' that results from '*the interplay of individual efforts, available resources, and contextual and structural factors as they come together in particular ... unique situations*' (Biesta and Tedder, 2007, p 137). Therefore, agency is not something people either possess or don't possess, but is something they can develop in transaction with their situation.

Agential concepts include self-efficacy, locus-of-control, autonomy and self-reliance. Self-efficacy is the belief individuals hold about their ability to achieve desired outcomes (Huberman, 1989), which determines how opportunities are perceived, how choices are made, and the effort and persistence made. Locus-of-control relates to a person's perception of internal control over external conditions (Rotter, 1966). When individuals perceive outcomes to be dependent on or influenced by their own skill or efforts, they have a greater sense of power and influence. Conversely, when individuals perceive their own skills and efforts have little impact on outcomes, their sense of powerlessness and ineffectiveness increases. For this reason, individuals '*will act differently in different contexts and at different times depending on how they perceive [their] locus-of-control*' (Pantic, 2015, p 768). Different arrangements and levels of authority can therefore influence our sense of control and effectiveness as practitioners. Autonomy is concerned with independent practice, where professionals self-govern their work and are accountable for the informed but independent decisions they make. Self-reliance is linked to this, as it denotes reliance on one's own capabilities, judgement or resources, with opportunities to exercise these being shown to develop identity and agency (see Chapter 10).

Resilience and confidence are concepts that also interact with agency. One definition of resilience is the ability to cope with and recover from adversity and change (Gu, 2016). This is an important resource for managing moral stress such as that created by role-identity conflict (Callero, 1985), with a balance between resignation and resistance being important. Confidence, which is a feeling of assurance or certainty, especially in oneself and one's capabilities, but also in other people or things, makes an important contribution, and strong professional agency has been found to:

- be central to identity development;
- foster work-related learning, commitment and well-being;
- be an important factor in change and development; and
- contribute to resilience and retention.

Time to consider 🗨

»   Think of a time you have felt empowered to action – what happened as a result?

»   Think of a time you have felt disempowered – what factors made you feel that way?

»   In contrast, what factors increase your agency?

Voice

Voice is significant to agency and change (Archer, 2000; Emirbayer and Mische, 1998). As a verb, voice means expressing something in words, for example 'she voiced her views'. As a noun it refers to a particular opinion or attitude, for example 'a dissenting voice' that needs to be listened to or granted a hearing.

Listening and responding to the voices of children and families are central to legislation, policy and practice (Unicef, nd; Children and Families Act, 2014; DfE and DoH, 2015; NSPCC, nd). Lundy (2007) proposed that four key elements are required for effective child voice: space (the opportunity to express a view); voice (individuals must be facilitated to express their views); audience (the view must be listened to); and influence (the view must be acted on, as appropriate).

These elements are also essential for practitioner voice, which sometimes *'may be frail, especially among those with little power'* (Holland et al, 1998, p 5). The creation of 'spaces' where practitioners can actively participate and contribute to policy and practice is essential, as are safe places through which concerns can be voiced. Sisson (2016) identifies risks associated with asserting one's voice against dominant discourses, which can include social isolation from colleagues, increased surveillance and even loss of job. Certainly, audience and influence vary, with professionals who hold 'higher' professional knowledge and status (eg paediatricians or educational psychologists) being respected and responded to more than practitioners who see the child, family and their environment, daily.

Critical question ❓

»   Pre-pandemic practitioner voices may have focused on improving resources to support existing organisation and systems rather than on significant changes (Warnes et al, 2021) whereas the focus of pandemic voices were health and safety, crisis management and advocacy (Clarke and Done, 2021). What do you think 'post' pandemic voices should focus on?

Spotlight on new debates

So far, the contribution of identity, agency and voice to practice has been explored. This section considers how these are enabled or constricted in practice. Bio-ecological systems theory (Bronfenbrenner, 1982) proposes macrosystem or institutional factors, such as socio-political culture and legislation, and exosystem or organisational factors, such as policy, ethos and funding, interact with a persons' microsystem or individual circumstances through the mesosystem. There can be a dynamic, bidirectional influence between these systems (Hayes et al, 2017). Figure 1.1 therefore synthesises Bronfenbrenner's bio-ecological systems with identity and agency to illustrate the effect influences in your ecological systems can have on your real and ideal identities, and on your agency.

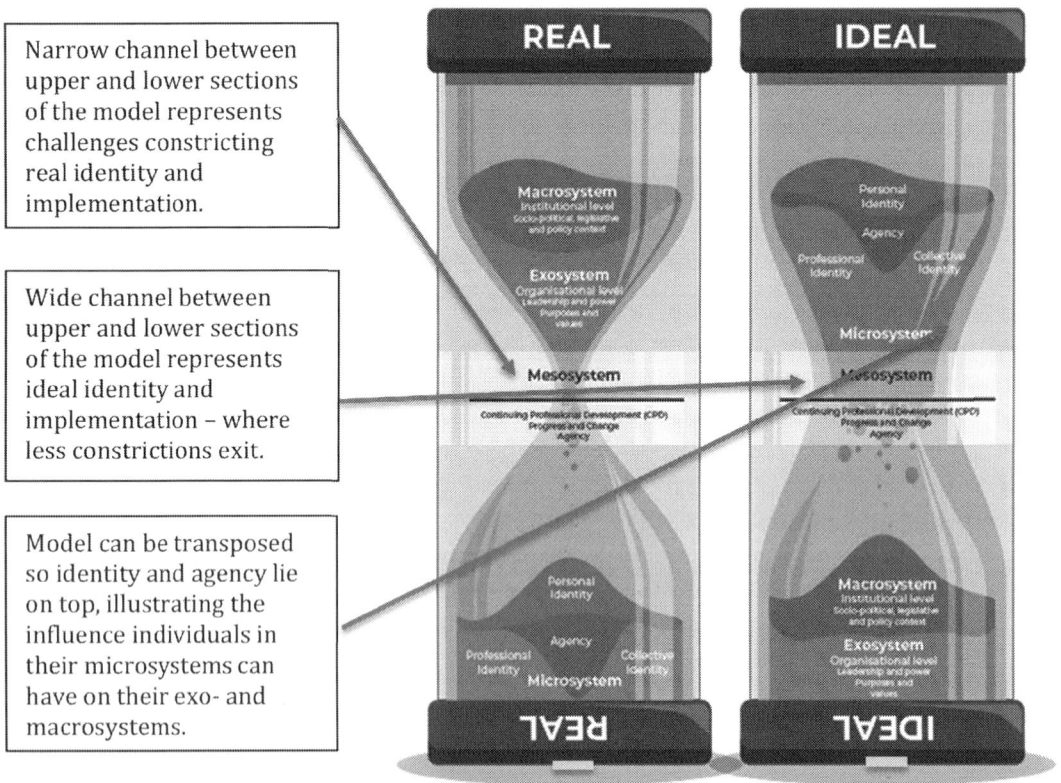

Narrow channel between upper and lower sections of the model represents challenges constricting real identity and implementation.

Wide channel between upper and lower sections of the model represents ideal identity and implementation – where less constrictions exit.

Model can be transposed so identity and agency lie on top, illustrating the influence individuals in their microsystems can have on their exo- and macrosystems.

Figure 1.1 *Diagram of real and ideal identity and agency, linked to Bronfenbrenner's ecological systems theory (Richards, 2019)*

In Figure 1.1, Bronfenbrenner's systems are represented within the halves of the sand timer to demonstrate that movement and influence occur between them. Macrosystem (institutional level) and exosystem influences (organisational level) are contained in one half of the sand timer since influences at these levels affect how practitioners carry out their responsibilities. These have both commonalities (legislation and policy) and variances depending on the values, purpose and power of leaders and setting ethos. The other half of the sand timer represents the microsystem of practitioners working within these systems. Detail about identity has been added to the microsystem as well as agency as self-formation (Holland et al, 1998). The chronosystem is implied rather than specifically labelled in the model, since it is a sand timer.

The two halves of the sand timer are connected via the mesosystem. The mesosystem in Figure 1.1 includes continuing professional development (CPD) opportunities, the capacity to influence change and affect progress, and effectual agency (Korsgaard, 2009). The left-hand sand timer has a narrowed channel between the macro- and exosystems and the microsystem, which represents the constrictions that often exist in reality. That is, where mismatches and/or constrictions exist between practice/work and ethos/approach, the reality can be practitioners whose agency is dampened. This contrasts with the right-hand sand timer which has a wider, more open channel between the microsystem and the macro and exosystems, thus representing ideal practice. That is, where a good match between practice/work and ethos/approach exists, the individual is more able to realise their ideal identity, agency and voice to effect change at institutional (macro) and organisational (exo) levels.

Time to consider ☁

» Think about an occasion when you needed to speak out or act in practice, and were you able to do so?

» What enabled you to do so? What constricted you from doing so?

» What areas of the institutional (macro) and organisational (exo) factors present in your setting are you able to influence?

» What areas do you feel less able to influence and why?

Developing your identity, agency and voice

Factors that enable or constrict real and ideal identity, agency and voice have been considered. This section considers practitioner attributes and features associated with effective practice (Figure 1.2), then suggests how individual practitioners can empower their agency (Figure 1.3).

Figure 1.2 depicts attributes of helpful, effective practitioners which emerged from research undertaken with 15 SENCos working in the early years or primary phase of education (Richards, 2019). Participants were asked to compare and contrast professionals whose practice they perceived to be helpful or unhelpful, before identifying how close these professionals were to their idea of effective practice. The professionals identified by participants included a range of roles across education, health and care, for example, educational psychologists, EHCP caseworkers, speech and language therapists, paediatricians, social workers and teachers.

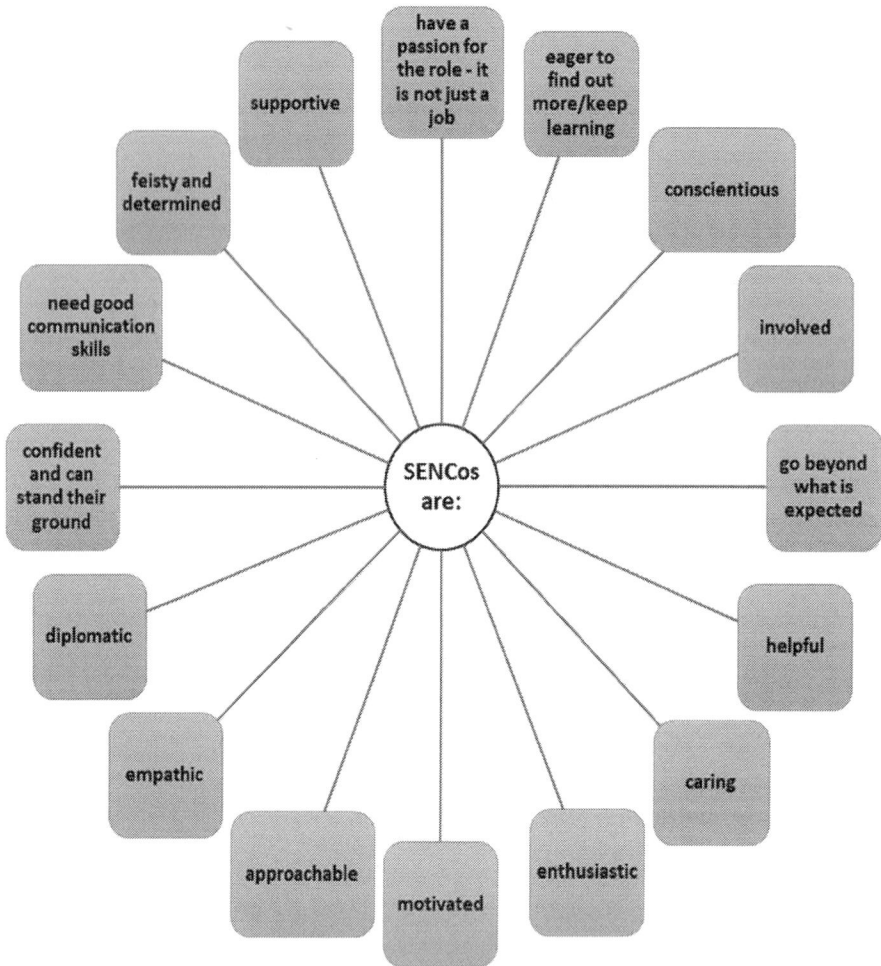

The attributes that emerged from the data (Figure 1.2) are therefore applicable to practitioners supporting children and families across a range or roles.

Figure 1.2 *Attributes of helpful, effective SENCos (Richards, 2019)*

Time to consider 💭

» Think about which attributes you already hold?

» Are there any other attributes you would like to add?

» Which attributes would you like to focus upon as you develop your professional skills?

The case study below will support you to think about why the attributes of helpful, effective practitioners are important.

CASE STUDY ☻

Hamida, 44, learning support practitioner

I had always had a thirst for education and as a young child had dreams of walking with giants someday ... However, I soon realised the views I had on education differed greatly from those of my parents and my community. It was simple – education was for males.

I struggled but accepted this as my only option so I found myself married by my late teens in the unpaid, unappreciated and repetitive role of a housewife. By 28 I had five children, controlling in-laws and a partner who was diagnosed with paranoid schizophrenia. Stating it mildly, life was extremely tough and challenging, and writing this brought back distressing memories. Life was slowly destroying me from the inside but my children needed me so I had to stay strong. However, my dreams and aspirations, coupled with hope, gave me the will to carry on.

Plucking up the courage to ask my children's headteacher for a voluntary position was a brave move as it went against the wishes of specific individuals in my life, but I ignored these protests and persevered as I needed something for myself. Beautiful souls nurtured me and before long I had enrolled in college. I completed my maths qualification in addition to my levels 2 and 3 Supporting Teaching and Learning NVQ. Things progressed further. I juggled work, family and study and completed my Foundation Degree, gaining recognition from college and university (I am so proud of my Outstanding Academic Achievement Award and trophy!). Then, in 2020, I completed my BA and achieved a first-class degree with honours from the University of Worcester.

Although I do not yet have an official role, I believe education has considerably altered my status. Not only do women from my community approach me for advice but I have regular supportive conversations with women from an array of backgrounds and races. They know I am always happy to help on a personal and professional level and the respect and admiration I receive from these souls are indescribably unique. I have inspired many women to undertake learning and provided reassurance and support and this is an area where I feel that I have been an agent of change. As a result, many have started volunteering, some have secured small jobs and a great number have qualified as teaching assistants.

The attitudes of my community are slowly changing too. Girls are being supported, are encouraged to complete education and are given choices. I feel mindsets are altering slowly from fixed to growth and I feel satisfied that I have played a part in this. I will always be grateful to CN for allowing me to volunteer in her setting (THANK YOU!), and I consider myself a prime example of the idea that through guidance and effort intellectual abilities can increase (Dweck, 1999).

Time to consider 💭

» Reflect on Hamida's account. What impression has it made on you?

» Identify attributes that Hamida demonstrates.

» In what areas of your life might you be able to be an agent of change and what attributes will you need?

Contexts both constrain and enable practice (see Figure 1.1), but are not, of themselves, '*the point of origin of agentic possibilities*' (Emirbayer and Mische, 1998, p 974). Instead, agentic possibilities reside at the level of self. Figure 1.3 therefore suggests how individual practitioners can empower their agency and so influence outcomes for the children and families they work with.

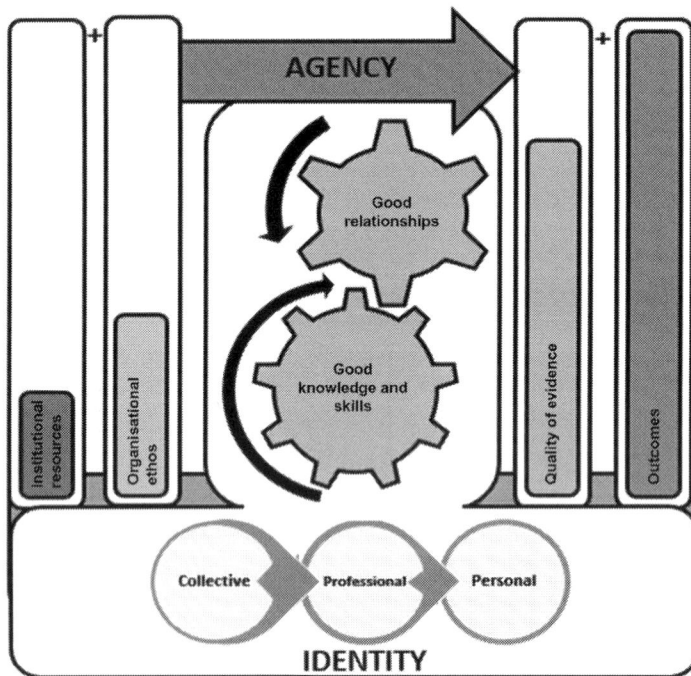

Figure 1.3 *Strong agentic influence on evidence and outcomes (where relationships and knowledge and skills are good) (Richards, 2019)*

Figure 1.3 shows identity (collective, professional and personal) as the base on which agency rests. This is because it is through individuals that organisations act, meaning that the collective, professional and personal identity of practitioners underlie and contribute to systemic change. This means that while the institutional resources available (far left column), and organisational ethos (inner left column) are important, in fact the quality of evidence and outcomes (depicted in the two columns to the right of agency) can be raised by agents who have established good working relationships and who hold good knowledge and skills. This is because practitioner power is most active when agents work with other agents. Interpersonal interactions and relationships are key for collaboration and for acting with other agents. Indeed, the presence and strength of the relationships (see the cog in the centre of the diagram) and networks practitioners hold with key groups of people, including professionals and caseworkers, setting staff, families, children and young people, and with their own peers and support network are central to person-centred, multi-professional care. Relationships are therefore a core area that practitioners and their settings should foreground.

Networks and connections also provide sources of support and information, since collaborative practice provides opportunities to engage with others, to include engaging with their knowledge and skills, and to critically consider different options. Figure 1.3 therefore also suggests that knowledge (including knowledge of process, of developmental norms, of individual children and their circumstances) and skills (including interpersonal communication and liaison) are key factors in strong agency. Furthermore, collaboration and engaging with others' knowledge and skills will help develop your understanding of your specific child and family support role and will clarify how and what you can contribute (Anning et al, 2010). You should therefore recognise the contribution knowledge and skills make to informed practice and improved outcomes, which may mean embracing opportunities for online learning, forum and team meeting platforms, as progressed in the Covid-19 era.

Time to consider 💭

» Think honestly and critically about your current knowledge and skill set. Which aspects are strong? Which areas are less strong?

» Who or what might be able to help you develop knowledge and skills in these areas?

CASE STUDY 🔊

Monique, student welfare officer, comprehensive secondary school

I have been working in education for around five years, but I'm now at a point where I want to take my career in a specific direction. I have started studying and completed the first year of my degree. I am neurodiverse and have a passion for inclusion. The knowledge I have gained in my study so far has further fuelled this passion and given me a definitive idea of where I want to take my personal development and career. However, I have become increasingly frustrated with the culture in education and how 'dismissive' it can be towards those who 'don't fit the system'.

I find resistance to making reasonable adjustments the more frustrating element of this culture. While I get it can be difficult without endless pots of money and resources, one thing we can control is our attitude. Becoming fed up with dealing with inflexibility, I felt the need to challenge senior staff. Armed with more knowledge following subject reading, I became familiar with the Equality Act 2010 and other useful literature to support my passions which added weight to my points. I have stopped accepting the phrase 'It sets a precedent' – I challenge it with 'whatever happened to individuality and teaching future generations about embracing difference?'

→

However, I knew I needed support because I felt like I was fighting a losing battle, so I decided to approach somebody who I felt would listen, and I am certainly glad I did. This person was in a senior position and offered me much needed reassurance and told me the reason I felt like this was because I care. All I need to do is remain objective, use my knowledge gained throughout study and this will enable me to strive for the best for the young people, their families, my institution and also the wider education sector, reducing reactive practice and promoting proactive approaches and inclusive culture all round.

Time to consider ☁

» How is Monique using her knowledge to empower her agency?

» What lessons can you take from this for your own practice?

» Identify a professional relationship that supports and enhances your practice. What features make this so helpful?

Chapter summary 🗓

Our identities are multifaceted (personal, professional and collective) and inform our actions. Although our power to act and speak out can vary, where constraints exist, for example in resources and setting ethos, practitioners can still enhance their potential to exercise agency and voice. Change and betterment for the children and families with whom we work can be empowered when practitioners build their held knowledge, skills and relationships, since as Kelly (1955, p 15) wrote:

> there are always some alternative constructions available to choose among in dealing with the world. No one needs to paint himself (sic) into a corner; no one needs to be completely hemmed in by circumstances; no one needs to be the victim of this biography.

My hope is you prove the power of this in your own practice.

Further reading 📖

Hayes, N, O'Toole, L and Halpenny, A M (2017) *Introducing Bronfenbrenner: A Guide for Practitioners and Students in Early Years Education.* Oxford: Routledge.

• This book explores the bidirectional relationship between children and their environments. Although aimed at early years, the core theory is relevant to all other age groups.

Melling, A and Pilkington, R (2018) *Paulo Freire and Transformative Education: Changing Lives and Transforming Communities.* London: Palgrave Macmillan.

• Freire believed in the possibility of change, emphasising the power of education to transform. Part 2 is especially relevant.

References

Anning, A, Cottrell, D, Frost, N, Green, J and Robinson, M (2010) *Developing Multi-professional Teamwork for Integrated Children's Services*. Buckingham: Open University Press.

Archer, M (2000) *Being Human: The Problem of Agency*. Cambridge: Cambridge University Press.

Ball, D (1972) Self and Identity in the Context of Deviance: The Case of Criminal Abortion. In Scott, R and Douglas, J (eds) *Theoretical Perspectives on Deviance*. New York: Basic Books.

Berardi, F (2017) *Futurability: The Age of Impotence and the Horizon of Possibility*. London: Verso.

Biesta, G, Priestley, M and Robinson, S (2016) The Role of Beliefs in Teacher Agency. *Teachers and Teaching: theory and practice*, 21(6): 624–40.

Biesta, G and Tedder, M (2007) Agency and Learning in the Lifecourse: Towards an Ecological Perspective. *Studies in the Education of Adults*, 39(2): 132–49.

Bourdieu, P (2002) Habitus. In Hillier, J and Rooksby, E (eds) *Habitus: A Sense of Place*. Aldershot: Ashgate.

Bronfenbrenner, U (1982) Ecological Systems Theory. In Vasta, R (ed) *Annals of Child Development. Six Theories of Child Development: Revised Formulations and Current Issues*. London: Jessica Kingsley.

Callero, P L (1985) Role-identity Salience. *Social Psychology Quarterly*, 48(3): 203–15.

Children and Families Act (2014). [online] Available at: www.legislation.gov.uk/ukpga/2014/6/contents/enacted (accessed 22 June 2021).

Clarke, A L and Done, E J (2021) Balancing Pressures for SENCos as Managers, Leaders and Advocates in the Emerging Context of the Covid-19 Pandemic. *British Journal of Special Education*. doi: 10.1111/1467-8578.12353.

Cooley, C H (1902) *Human Nature and the Social Order*. New York: Schocken Books.

DfE and DoH (Department for Education and Department of Health) (2015) *Special educational needs and disability code of practice: 0 to 25 years*. [online] Available at: www.gov.uk/government/publications/send-code-of-practice-0-to-25 (accessed 22 June 2021).

Emirbayer, M and Mische, A (1998) 'What Is Agency?'. *American Journal of Sociology*, 103(4): 962–1023. doi: 10.1086/231294.

Erikson, E H (1959) *Identity and the Life Cycle*. New York: Norton.

Gu, Q (2016) The role of Relational Resilience in Teacher's Career-long Commitment and Effectiveness. *Teachers and Teaching: Theory and Practice*, 20(5): 502–29.

Holland, D, Lachicotte, W, Skinner, D and Cain, C (1998) *Identity and Agency in Cultural Worlds*. Cambridge, MA: Harvard University Press.

Huberman, M (1989) The Professional Life Cycle of Teachers. *Teachers College Record*, 91(1): 31–57.

Illeris, K (2014) Transformative Learning and Identity. *Journal of Transformative Education*, 12(1): 148–63.

Isaksson, J and Lindqvist, R (2015) 'What Is the Meaning of Special Education?' Problem Representations in Swedish Policy Documents: Late 1970s – 2014. *European Journal of Special Needs Education*, 30(1): 122–37. doi: 10.1080/08856257.2014.964920.

Jenkins, R (2004) *Social Identity*. London: Routledge.

Jo, S, H (2014) Teacher Commitment: Exploring Associations with Relationships and Emotions. *Teaching and Teacher Education*, 43: 120–30.

Kelly, G A (1955) *The Psychology of Personal Constructs Volumes 1 and 2*. New York: Norton.

Korsgaard, C M (2009) *Self-constitution: Agency, Identity, and Integrity*. Oxford: Oxford University Press.

Lundy, L (2007) 'Voice' Is Not Enough: Conceptualising Article 12 of the United Nations Convention on the Rights of the Child. *British Educational Research Journal*, 33(6): 927–42.

Mead, G H (1934) Mind, Self and Society: From the Standpoint of a Social Behaviourist. Edited with Morris, C W. Chicago: University of Chicago Press.

Meyer, E and Lees, A (2013) Learning to Collaborate: An Application of Activity Theory to Interprofessional Learning across Children's Services. *Social Work Education*, 32(4): 662–84.

Mollenhauer, K (2014) *Forgotten Connections: On Culture and Upbringing*. Edited and translated by Friesen, N. London: Routledge.

NSPCC (nd) Case Reviews. [online] Available at: https://learning.nspcc.org.uk/case-reviews (accessed 22 June 2021).

Pantic, N (2015) A Model for Study of Teacher Agency for Social Justice. *Teachers and Teaching: Theory and Practice*, 21(6): 759–78.

Phillips, S P and Dalgarno, N (2017) Professionalism, Professionalization, Expertise and Compassion: A Qualitative Study of Medical Residents. *BMC Medical Education*, 17(21): 1–7.

Pyhältö, K, Pietarinen, J and Soini, T (2015) Teachers' Professional Agency and Learning – from Adaption to Active Modification in the Teacher Community. *Teachers and Teaching: Theory and Practice*, 21(6): 811–30.

Richards, H (2019) *Special Educational Needs Co-ordinator perceptions of practice and potential: investigating education and health care plan implementation in early years and primary education*. PhD thesis. [online] Available at: http://eprints.worc.ac.uk/9919/ (accessed 22 June 2021).

Roldàn, L I (1992) From the Barrio to the Academy: Revelations of a Mexican American 'Scholarship Girl'. *New Directions for Community Colleges*, 80, 55–64. [online] Available at: https://laurare ndonnet.files.wordpress.com/2018/07/from-barrio.pdf (accessed 19 July 2021).

Rotter, J B (1966) Generalized Expectancies for Internal versus External Control of Reinforcement. *Psychological Monographs: General and Applied*, 80(1): 1–28.

Sisson, J H (2016) The Significance of Critical Incidents and Voice to Identity and Agency. *Teachers and Teaching*, 22(6): 670–82.

Taylor, C (1985) *Human agency and Language*. Cambridge: Cambridge University Press.

Unicef (nd) United Nations Convention on the Rights of the Child. [online] Available at: www.unicef.org.uk/what-we-do/un-convention-child-rights/ (accessed 22 June 2021).

Vähäsantanen, K (2015) Professional Agency in the Stream of Change: Understanding Educational Change and Teachers' Professional Identities. *Teaching and Teacher Education*, 47: 1–12.

Van de Putte, I, De Shauwer, E, Van Hove, G and Davies, B (2017) Rethinking Agency as an Assemblage from Change Management to Collaborative Work. *International Journal of Inclusive Education*, 22(8): 885–901.

Warnes, E, Done, E J and Knowler, H (2021) Mainstream Teachers' Concerns about Inclusive Education for Children with Special Educational Needs and Disability in England under Pre-pandemic Conditions. *Journal of Research in Special Educational Needs*. https://doi.org/10.1111/1471-3802.12525

2 Empowering reflective practice

HAZEL RICHARDS AND MICHELLE MALOMO

What do we mean by reflection?

Solutions and possibilities

How reflection is traditionally used

Empowering reflective practice

What is my identity, and what are my attributes, values and beliefs?

The importance of self-awareness

Chapter objectives ◎

This chapter considers how you can use reflection to develop your professional identity and maintain your resilience. The chapter:

- uses theory to build your understanding of what is meant by the term 'reflection';

- explores some of the ways reflection has been traditionally applied;

- considers new research and debates in the development of a personal approach to reflection;

- proposes how you can use the power of reflection to build your confidence and empower your practice.

Critical questions ⑦

»   What do you already know about reflection?

»   When you do something well in practice, how do you celebrate it?

»   How else do you currently use reflection?

Introduction

Work with children and their families involves diverse, novel and sometimes challenging situations where there is no 'off the shelf' solution. Instead, decisions about appropriate responses and courses of action must be reached by critically and objectively considering multiple perspectives and issues. As authors, our practice within diverse parts of the sector means we have experienced several approaches to, and perspectives of, reflection. The aim of this chapter is, therefore, to explore different ways you might reflect and help you find a personally meaningful approach by investigating theory and recent developments.

What do we mean by 'reflection'?

An exact answer to this question may not be possible because of varying perspectives and experiences, as mentioned above. This section therefore summarises some main theorists who have contributed to the development of reflection over the last 100 years, and explores meanings of the term 'reflection', so as to build your understanding and help you recognise your own stance, before new and emerging ways of thinking are considered later in the chapter.

Our lived experiences shape our worldviews (Dewey 1933, 1938, 1958) and transactions between individuals and their environments and experiences shape each person's responses and actions (Dewey and Bentley, 1949). Schön (1983) presents the connection between the environment where experiences occur and the reflective process, explaining that we reflect both during and after experiences. He described these two types of reflection as 'reflection-in-action' and 'reflection-on-action'. Table 2.1 summarises the key differences between these:

Table 2.1 *Reflecting-in-action and reflecting-on-action*

Reflection-**in**-action	Reflecting-**on**-action
• Conducted while the event is still happening.	• Happens after an event.
• 'Thinking on your feet' that results in 'experimentation' as a kind of action.	• Allows a professional to analyse the event and reframe a problematic situation.
• Develops with practice to become a way of 'being'.	• Results in continual review and repositioning in-order-to effect change and improvement.

Source: Schön (1983).

While there can be more time to reflect after an event, Schön (1983) suggested practitioners use these two types of reflection interactively, because they do not separate thinking from doing. There may have been times when you have had to apply this responsive in-the-moment approach (which can help us develop confidence in our own abilities and skills). Equally, we also need times when we step back and reframe our thinking before we make a response. Mezirow (1998, p 185) described reflection as a *'turning back'* on, or pondering an experience. He compared this with critical reflection, which has the potential to change our assumptions or frame of reference, as this more interrogative process requires us to bring to awareness, then examine and weigh up the significant factors in an experience, including our reasons for responding in the way we did.

Reflection is often considered to be subjective although Siegal (1988) states critical reflection is principled thinking in that ideally it is impartial, consistent and systematic. Its purpose is to allow us to identify, evaluate and adapt our responses, though this is not always easy. Work with children and their families involves emotion and will always mean collaborating with those who hold their own set of values. Brookfield's (1995) theory helps us to step back and see things through other eyes (like the balcony approach proposed by Paige-Smith and Craft, 2011). Brookfield (1995, p 61) suggests we must be aware of our own interpretive filters since we all hold perceptual frameworks that determine how we construe our experiences, proposing '*the only way we can become aware of our assumptions, particularly ones we've missed or been unaware of, is to view what we do through the equivalent of the side mirrors in the clothing booth*'. He suggests there are four key mirrors/lenses to consider as we critically reflect (see Table 2.2).

Table 2.2 The four lenses of critical reflection

Autobiographical lens	Student lens	Colleagues/peers lens	Theoretical lens
Our personal viewpoint, which can be restricted due to our experience and which will contain 'blind spots'.	Requires us to listen to the voice, priorities and preferences of those most closely and significantly affected by our practice.	Discussing and debating our experiences with others to reveal alternative ways to approach shared experiences or problems.	Theory can make '*explicit something you've been sensing*' or state '*publicly what you've suspected privately*'. It can also '*unsettle the groupthink arising from cultural norms*', and so provides a means of framing/re-framing your thinking (pp 73–4).

Source: Adapted from Brookfield (1995).

Reflection, therefore, is undertaken both during and after experiences and requires us to consider multiple perspectives. But how do we actually 'do' it and how might it empower us? Ghaye et al (2008, p 361) propose reflection is a means of developing appreciative insight, by helping us understand '*the root causes of success and sustaining strengths-based discourses*'. They suggest participatory and appreciative action and reflection (PAAR) should not only allow us to consider 'problems' we need to 'fix'. Rather, it should also be about understanding which aspects of our life and work are successful, and how '*joyful and celebratory aspects of practice can be further amplified and made more consistent*' (p 362). Reflection therefore involves recognising and playing to our strengths, as well as scoping and identifying approaches to meet the challenges.

Some theorists propose reflection is a continuous process. For example, Kolb's (1984) cycle of experiential learning involves four stages (see Figure 2.1).

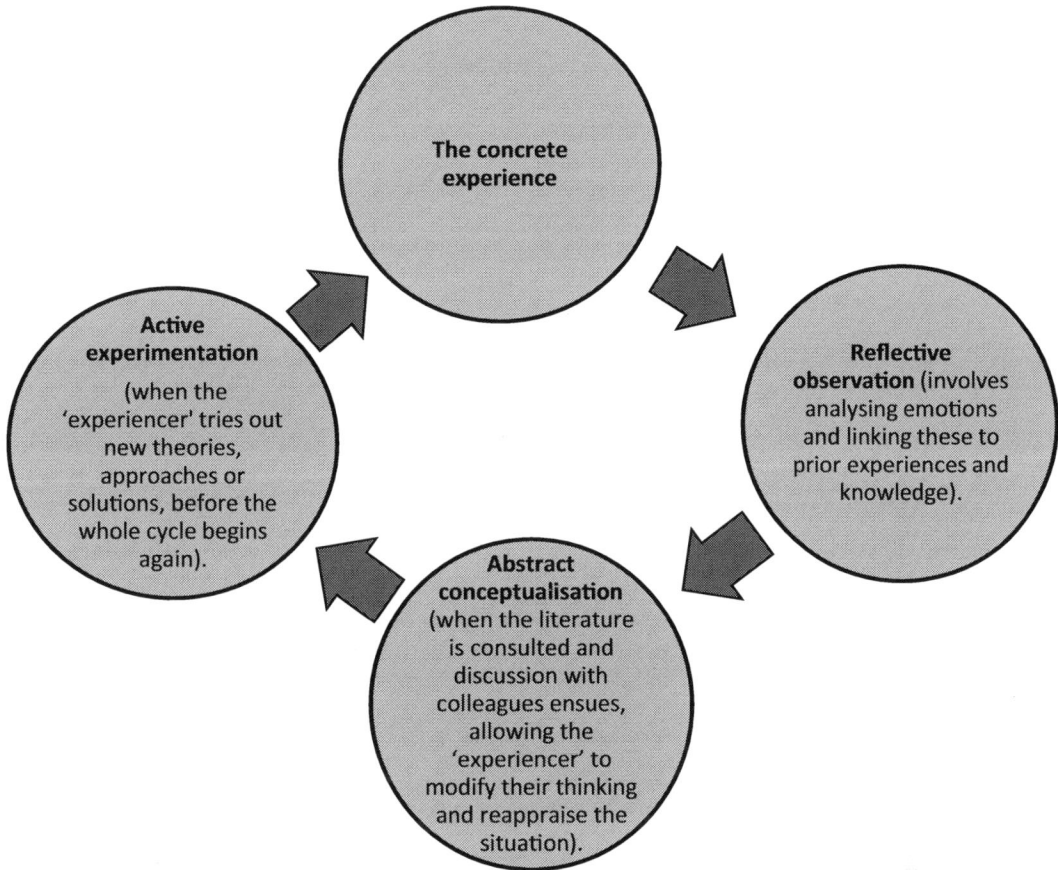

Figure 2.1 *Adapted from Kolb's (1984) cycle of experiential learning*

This has similarities to the assess-plan-do-review cycle applied to identify and provide support needed by students with Special Educational Needs and Disabilities (SEND), and to the early years HighScope Approach (HighScope, nd), though is simpler than Gibb's (1988) reflective cycle, which consists of six stages (event description; exploring feelings; evaluating positive and challenging aspects of the experience; analysing the situation to identify impact; consulting literature and colleagues to reach a conclusion to; formulate an action plan). What is common to each model is recognition of the emotional response and evaluation.

These models (Kolb, assess-plan-do-review, HighScope, Gibbs) are all single-loop reflective cycles. In contrast, in double-loop cycles (Argyris and Schön, 1974, 1978) the individual does not merely seek alternative actions or plans but also reflects on their values and beliefs. Double-loop reflection therefore, involves deeper interrogation of sometimes subconscious and ethical stances, so corresponds with Brookfield's autobiographical lens. Furthermore, Argyris and Schön (1974, 1978) argue individuals have a subconscious tendency to continue responding in a certain way, due to desires to keep other variables such as cost, stress and confidence within acceptable personal limits (Redmond, 2017), but double-loop reflection encourages us to change predictable responses by recognising and modifying the beliefs and values directing them (see Figure 2.2).

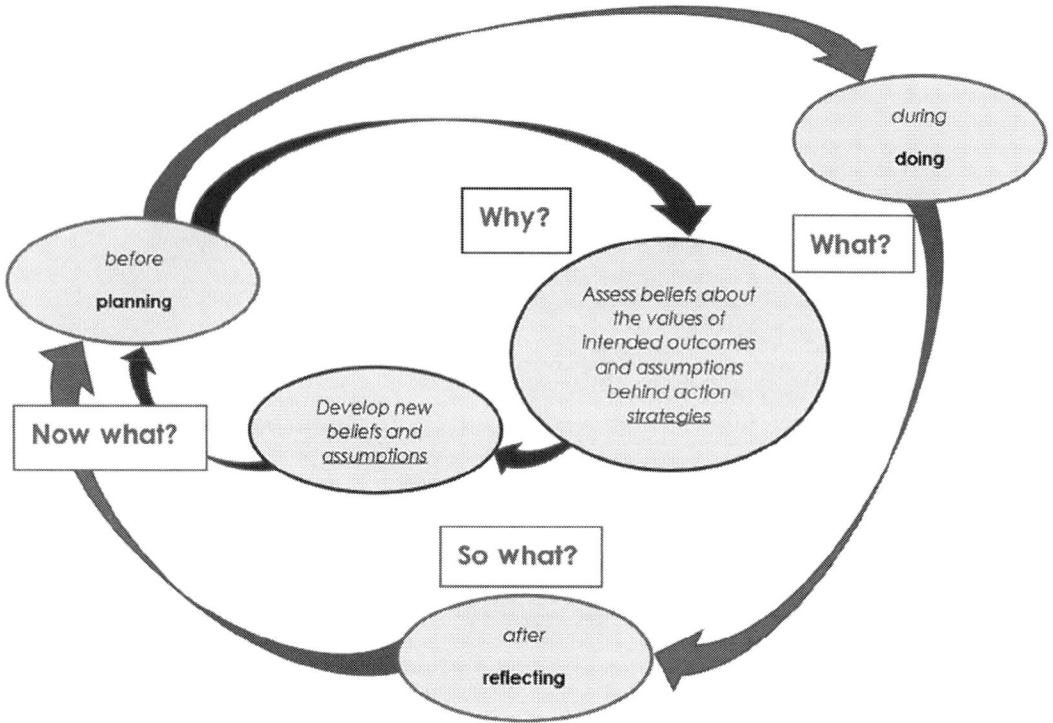

Figure 2.2 *Double-loop reflection, adapted from Argyris and Schön (1974, 1978)*

By making explicit the variables shaping your actions, double-loop reflection can therefore help you to avoid repeating ineffective actions. It is also an important step in allowing you to interrogate and reframe your thinking about a given experience, which can free you to consider and explore innovative and creative responses to problematic and/or persistent challenges.

Time to consider ☁

How might these historically accepted discourses apply to your own practice and learning?

»   Identify an experience from your own life or practice that had a significant influence on your education or career (Dewey).

»   Recognise a time when you had to think quickly or react 'on your feet', and how you viewed this action after the event (Schön).

»   Think back on a recent experience: from your own perspective and from the perspective of the child and family, your colleagues and using knowledge you have accrued in your studies. What is different about each viewpoint? (Brookfield).

> » Is there an area of your practice or life where you repeatedly respond in a particular way, even though this may be ineffective? Ponder deeply and see if you can identify the factors that make you do this. Can you identify anything you could change, despite the presence of these factors? (Argyris and Schön).

How reflection is traditionally used

Reflection has been written about extensively and its very nature means perspectives and approaches evolve. Traditionally used to develop and improve praxis, defined by Reed (2010, p 25) as *'the integration of practice, experience, interpretive reasoning and reflection applied towards purposeful action'*, reflective practice applies a structured process or cycle to identify how to address or improve problematical situations. However, if it lacks deep interrogation, practitioners are in danger of, at best, finding optimal ways of working within the constraints, or at worst, accommodating them (Adams, 2009). Moreover, although reflective practice responds to complexity, or what Schön (1987, p 3) describes as the *'swampy zones of practice involving uncertainty, uniqueness and value conflict'*, practitioners often need to make complex value judgements in-the-moment.

Ruch (2007) explores beyond reflection-**in**-action and reflection-**on**-action (Schön, 1983) (see Table 2.3), stating the challenge is not to privilege one model of reflection over another, but to keep them all in play.

Table 2.3 Ruch's (2007) models of reflection

Practical reflection	Critical reflection	Technical reflection	Process reflection
Reflecting on 'bottom-up'/from practice experience to develop knowledge and skills.	Reflecting on existing social conditions and structural forces to identify routes for change with a view to emancipation.	Privileging expert and external sources of knowledge in instrumental, problem-solving.	Focusing on conscious and unconscious aspects of practice and acknowledging the impact of the emotional nature of the work.

Holistic reflection, which recognises the reality and impact of the emotional elements of the work, is needed where the culture of 'always trying to be better' can feel like a hamster wheel, leaving limited time and energy to manage one's own feelings. We know work with children and families can require practitioners to suppress their own feelings in order to present an appropriate outward appearance (Williams, 2013), with Ferguson (2018) identifying that there are times when reflection is either limited or non-existent when practitioners defend themselves against the emotional impact and anxiety provoked by the work. Hochschild (2003) named the task of managing emotional demands involved with a job 'emotional labour' and considered the toll this can have on personal lives. The global pandemic has increased the loads, emotional and otherwise, placed on practitioners as well as blurring boundaries between home and work. Emotionally challenging work can also place demands on individual practitioners that conflict with their personal values and identity.

The definition of reflective practice as reflective activism (Hanson and Appleby, 2015) draws on Freire's (1973) argument for emancipation through critical consciousness of the world. The world has shifted seismically in response to the Covid-19 pandemic; for instance, workers involved with children and their families became 'key-workers' despite being of low status materially and hierarchically, and the complexity and emotional load of their work increased at the same time as challenges at home. Reflection can help navigate such changes, with effective reflective practitioners holding thorough understandings of themselves, including of the values and moral purposes underlying their practice and knowledge of their working contexts (Leitch and Day, 2000). Such awareness is more essential than ever as we work with those who have experienced increased privations, mental health and well-being issues. Ixer (2016) asks whether reflection is skills or values based, proposing the ability to self-evaluate has the power to become transformative and emancipatory. The reality is, dilemmas thrown up in practice can demand critical and moral analysis, as Grace's case study illustrates.

CASE STUDY 🖐

Grace, newly qualified children's nurse, working on a general children's ward

I started work in May 2020, straight after handing in my thesis, and before my 21st birthday. My initial months of practice therefore involved lots of emotional labour due to the high number of children admitted for safeguarding and/or mental health issues, though I found one case particularly challenging.

During a night shift I was assigned an eight week-old baby with breathing difficulties. This baby had some safeguarding issues, so parents did not visit at all. She required hourly observations and had very high blood pressure, which was more dangerous in her case as she required surgery for a heart issue. Uncontrolled blood pressure is always a serious sign in infants, so I escalated my unease to the doctors several times. However, they were not concerned. The baby was very distressed and due to her being on her own, we did not know how parents settled her. Between about 1am and 5am I could not leave her for a second as she would become very unsettled, and her oxygen saturation levels kept dipping. Still the doctors did not listen to my concerns until nearly 5am, when they finally recognised the seriousness and contacted the Children's Hospital for advice as we could not keep on top of her oxygen saturations and blood pressure, and we could not settle her. By this stage I was exhausted and fed up as I felt I was trying all I could but at the same time I felt I was not doing enough. Eventually, the nurse-in-charge came in and gave the baby a sedative medication to help her sleep as advised by the Children's Hospital, helping her finally settle for the remaining three and a half hours of my 12.5-hour shift.

The nurse-in-charge could tell something was wrong with me and called me into the office at the end of my shift to find out. At this stage I was exhausted and could not control my emotions and I just burst into tears as I felt I had spent hours trying to get the doctors to listen and attempting to settle her, and as a newly qualified nurse I felt I had not done enough. The nurse-in-charge helped me to reflect by looking at events as they had developed through the night which helped me to understand I had done everything I could have done. However, it can be very frustrating when doctors do not listen to nurses, despite them being the ones that are with the patients all the time. I recognise that my drive home from work provides an opportunity to reflect on your shift and the cases encountered, so on the way home, I reflected again on the night and thought about my feelings of frustration and disempowerment. Once I had got home and had some sleep, I woke to find many of my colleagues had messaged me to check I was doing alright and to send me words of encouragement, which helped my confidence and made me feel a bit better.

Critical questions ⑦

»   What aspects of emotional labour did you identify in Grace's reflection?

»   Now think about the emotional labour involved in your work – what impact could it have on you?

»   Identify a time when you have defended yourself against emotional impact and anxiety by consciously not reflecting? How did you manage this instead?

»   Reflect on an experience from your own practice that involved complexities and dilemmas – what values and emotions were involved and how did you manage these?

This chapter now explores new debates that prioritise self-awareness and guides you to think how you can develop your own personalised approach to reflection.

Spotlight on new debates

It is now important to consider what current research highlights, since this could expand your thinking about reflection and have an empowering effect on your reflective practice. Students come to their degree course with a diverse understanding of what reflection is. For some it is a new concept, for others it is part of day-to-day practice as they work. You may have already adopted one of the models of reflection as your approach. However, when reflection is adopted in this manner, and with the strain of practice, there may be a sense of what could be termed reflection fatigue. Reflective practice can then lose its power to develop your professional skills and identity. In addition, those who work within the sector have historically been marginalised and undervalued by society, which has influenced the practitioner's perceived professional identity (Papadopoulou, 2020) and may have limited reflection support mechanisms.

This societal perception needs to be acknowledged as you develop your reflective approach. However, do not restrict your mindset as you enter the process of reflection. Papadopoulou (2020) offers a further insight suggesting that it is important not to conform to the perceived expectations of the figured world but develop ways of changing it. Furthermore, she suggests that developing your professional identity involves a sense of self, of knowing your personal identity, attributes, values and beliefs, and the meaning that these bring. Connecting your reflective approach to who you are helps keep the reflective process grounded. Hanson and Appleby (2017) describe the process of reflection in this context as having a moral compass. Having worked with students as they explored the reflective process, they found it helpful to start with an identification of their identity, attributes, values and beliefs. Recognising these develops a conscious understanding of your personal moral compass. This is important because when placing yourself in practice, your moral compass collides with other practitioners, children and their families, community and society. Gutierrez and Vossoughi (2010) suggest that the ability to identify and see things from different vantage points supports our thinking about the contradictions that emerge in practice. This can support us in exploring and developing our initially held values, identity and beliefs, contributing to a professional identity that develops in an organic manner. Trodd and Dickerson (2019) state that supporting practitioners to develop their reflective skills creates a mechanism for acquiring this work-based knowledge. Indeed, they argue that such an approach engages the whole person and enhances a personal capacity for work-based learning that goes beyond merely fulfilling the needs of the workplace. Identifying your own moral compass will aid the reflective thinking process by offering a mechanism through which you can process your practice experiences, help you identify discontinuities and solutions, and reset your 'direction'.

To summarise, recent debates suggest that the reflective process needs to start with developing self-awareness of who you are and what you hold. This contrasts with the commonly held view of reflection as being about enhancing practice.

Developing your approach to self-reflection: solutions and possibilities

We now lead you through what could be termed a reflective discovery process to support you to develop confidence in the approach that you adopt. To start this reflective discovery, let's address the elephant in the room. Students can perceive that reflection is about identifying and focusing on the areas in which your practice is lacking, rather than celebrating successes within your work. Roberts (2020) addresses this, suggesting that you need to be kind to yourselves as you enter the reflective/change process, though she also acknowledges that reflection needs time and space, which is not always easy to secure within children and family work (Munro, 2017). Highlighting this at the start of the reflective discovery process is valuable. It means recognising practice is always changing and evolving and accepting you will not always get things right the first time. By approaching the reflective process with a sense of self-worth and kindness you begin at a place where the process empowers, rather than disempowers you. This may mean having a conversation with yourself and consciously approaching reflection from a position of kindness and being comfortable with not knowing. It is therefore important that any reflective approach you adopt is clear about your sense of who and what you are. Developing your personal moral compass can be a useful possibility. Use the 'Time to consider' below to support this thought process.

Time to consider

» Over the next week, notice and celebrate a positive experience or example of good practice.

» Think about how, when and why we use a compass. Consider how your compass can help recalibrate your direction when complexities and challenges create confusion.

» What could be important in your moral compass? Think about your identity, attributes, values and beliefs. You might want to record this in a reflective journal. It is useful to revisit this and acknowledge how this has developed as you make sense of emerging knowledge from work-based practice.

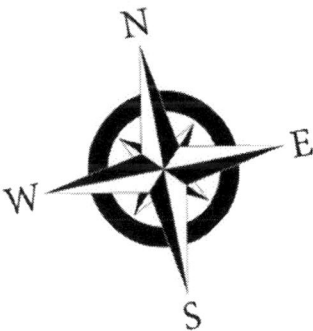

My identity (think about your personality traits)
For example, I am shy by nature which means that I dislike conflict.
My attributes (think about your skills and strengths)
For example, I am a planner and like to know what I am doing and always like to be prepared
My values
For example, I value listening to others and my thoughts being heard
My beliefs
For example, I believe in equality of opportunity

Figure 2.3 *Personal moral compass, Richards and Malomo (2021)*

Once you have an awareness of your moral compass, it is important that you recognise if you have adopted a theory to underpin your approach. Earlier in the chapter activities guided you through how you might use traditionally accepted theories. There are, however, emerging debates that explore the value of how we reflect. One approach is to value and understand the power of stories within the reflective process. Bolton and Delderfield

(2018, p 79) state that '*stories have themes which can inform the reader or listener about the culture, and society, about underlying, principles, assumptions about roles*'. Using narratives of shared experience has the power to unlock an understanding of who we are, what we value and what those with whom we work in practice value. This may appear complex; stories of an experience enable us to seek out cultures within our practice that can help explain why things are the way they are. Stories of practice can be captured within a journal. This can provide a sanctuary for the depositing of practice stories as we develop our knowledge. Journals can also provide a place of safety in which to document thoughts and emotions, and can help us to reflect on and consider emerging knowledge from our practice-based experiences. Best (1996) suggests that journals have a therapeutic value, in that identifying and documenting these thoughts and emotions help us make sense of ourselves within these experiences. During the Covid-19 pandemic, practitioners found themselves working within a society where everything they had known as 'normal' changed. Instead of being marginalised they became essential or key workers (DfE, 2021) and were given a status of an essential part of the country's recovery within government policy. This was almost unimaginable prior to the pandemic. Eigege and Kennedy (2021) state that we need to capture and value the narratives of practitioners living through this time. For example, Johnson (2020, p 208) recorded the following snapshot of their story during this period.

> *Reflecting on the past few months, I realise that at the onset of the pandemic I felt as if I were facing a huge jigsaw puzzle. The pieces of the world in which I work, and which once slotted neatly together were now in a jumbled heap and I had no idea how they would fit back together to make the familiar picture.*

The pandemic disturbed practice, providing opportunities for the sector to develop new ways of 'being' with children and their families. During this time there were constant changes to legislation and guidance that affected both the movement of practitioners within communities and the way in which they practised. It also enabled practice to be developed through new and innovative ways of engaging with children and their families. Disturbances within practice then can bring about unexpected change.

Time to consider 💭

» Having read the above snapshot, what can you perceive about Johnson's thoughts about her professional identity and practice?

» Have you ever experienced a time when you felt your practice was disturbed? How did this make you feel?

» Practice will not always be like a jigsaw puzzle that slots together and this is when we must be comfortable with not knowing. How might you respond if this happens within your practice?

» Read the case study below. How was Sally's practice disturbed and what helped her resolve this?

CASE STUDY ⟲

Sally, Higher Level Teaching Assistant and aspiring teacher, suburban primary school

Teaching through a global pandemic has significantly influenced my reflective practice, forcing me to understand the needs of the pupils in my class from a holistic perspective. The pandemic created uncertainty, from the logistics of how to teach remotely and engage pupils and parents, to concern over learning 'gaps' created through the absence of 'normal' teaching, to a complete shift in the assessment process.

In September 2020, my professional thinking was shaped in ways never previously considered. I was responsible for educating 30 little beings, which now included wearing face masks, sanitising routines, social distancing and reams of risk assessments. I needed to create an environment where my pupils felt – and were – safe, but not stifled; cared for, but not lacking in independence. This required lots of planning, but also extensive reflection – both reactionary while teaching and at the end of the school day, for example when I needed to mark books but felt uneasy about touching them. Reflection led to the implementation of 'live marking' along with 'whole class feedback'. I was also able to empower the children into marking their own work in particular lessons or tasks, which highlighted to them their own successes and next steps.

I recall being extremely anxious about the movement of the children in class: should they turn to track the speaker when the classroom environment is now forward-facing only? Did someone else just touch that rubber? Quick, sanitise! My (perhaps) irrational feelings were creeping into my teaching practice. Considering their perspective, here was a teacher new to them who looked like a rabbit in the headlights when a child happened to cough! I was also aware of the anxieties likely to be felt by the parents and carers and what they would be expecting from me with regard to 'lost learning'. Following discussion with colleagues, I realised my worries were not unique. Covid-preventative practices became embedded into the school day as if they were another block in the timetable and I made sure I knew my role in this new, strange world, and that the children knew theirs, which helped me manage my anxiety.

A key value at my setting is resilience, and the resilience of my pupils over this past year has been inspiring. I also feel proud of my own achievements. My periods of reflection continue to focus on my role: how can I teach this objective to the children, in a way they understand, to the level they require? Pandemic or no pandemic, reflection is always needed as we continue to strive to be the best practitioners that our pupils deserve.

Elfer and Wilson (2021) suggest that reflection has been presented as straightforward and unproblematic. This is a misconception. They suggest that any model of reflection must support practitioners to explore both conscious and unconscious emotion, then to discuss these. This is because in any personalised reflective approach, it is important to acknowledge that reflection is an emotive process, and so another form of emotional labour (Hochschild, 2003). Indeed, the demand of working within child and family work can be emotionally draining as well as rewarding (see Chapter 5). Just thinking about this contrast suggests that the reflective process will not be straightforward. Elfer and Wilson (2021) highlight that working within the sector involves deep human engagement which involves commitment and emotion, and they consider the value of work discussion as a method to support practitioner reflection. This involves practitioners coming together, being curious and exploring together what is not known about practice, but requires an emotionally supportive environment and culture of trust in addition to the other conditions Moon (2008) identified as enabling reflection. These include time and space, asking the right kind of questions, acknowledging the dangers of adherence to 'recipes' for reflection, developing habits of reflection, that is journaling, and challenging learners to integrate new learning into existing practice.

While this is similar to the clinical supervision integral to some professions, it may be a new concept to some. Elfer and Wilson (2021, p 2) also recognise that *'practitioners' own needs and vulnerabilities can be difficult to acknowledge but are an inevitable aspect of their humanity'*. This suggests that the range of emotions that practitioners feel is part of who they are. It is important then to have an awareness that reflection can make a significant contribution to sustaining our emotional balance in practice. For example, by having reflective pauses we can rebalance ourselves using reflection (see Figure 2.4).

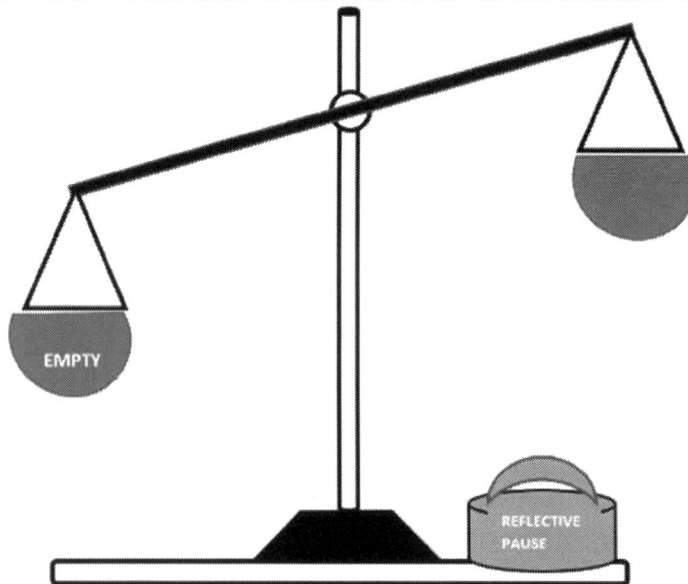

Figure 2.4 *Balancing the practice scales, Richards and Malomo (2021)*

Often, we can come to the reflective process almost running on empty and entering a reflective pause can be helpful in redressing the imbalance. This type of pause supports us in maintaining our own well-being and may involve journaling our thoughts or it may just involve taking a breath and gathering our thoughts. Chapter 3 considers self-care in further detail and you may find some of the strategies suggested there are also useful as part of your reflective pauses.

Chapter summary 📖

Reflection is a very personal process. Recent research emphasises the importance of sharing your thoughts and emotions about practice with those who work alongside you. The following questions therefore link to the key messages to enable you to identify and develop your own approach.

Critical questions ❓

» Identify what reflection methods worked best for you (eg Brookfield's lens). As a result of reading this chapter how will you add to and develop this?

» Having developed your thinking, for example by applying the compass model, what have you learned as a result about (a) your practice and (b) yourself?

» Thinking about the power of journaling as a reflect tool how could you use this to release you from the chain of reflection to the power of reflection as a way of being?

» Reflection requires you to identify the positive, not just the negative, and to be kind to yourself. Take time to identify what needs to be in your 'personal kindness kit'.

Further reading 📖

Bolton, G and Delderfield, R (2018) *Reflective Practice: Writing and Professional Development*. London: Sage.

• This book supports the discovery of your own reflective style and professional identity by exploring the power of reflective writing.

Hanson, K and Appleby, K (2015) 'Reflective Practice'. In Reed, M and Walker, R (eds) *A Critical Companion to Early Childhood* (pp 24–35). London: Sage.

• This chapter explores the idea of reflective activism, highlighting the need for an autobiographical lens.

References 📚

Adams, R (2009) 'Being a Critical Practitioner'. In Adams R, Dominelli, L and Payne, M (eds) *Critical Practice in Social Work* (2nd ed). Basingstoke: Palgrave-Macmillan.

Argyris, C and Schön, D (1974) *Theory in Practice: Increasing Personal Effectiveness*. San-Francisco: Jossey-Bass.

Argyris, C and Schön, D (1978) *Organizational Learning*. Reading, MA: Addison-Wesley Publishing Company.

Best, D (1996) On the Experience of Keeping a Therapeutic Journal while Training. *Therapeutic Communities*, 17(4): 293–301.

Bolton, G and Delderfield, R (2018) *Reflective Practice: Writing and Professional Development.* London: Sage.

Brookfield, S D (1987) *Developing Critical Thinkers: Challenging Adults to Explore Alternative Ways of Thinking and Acting.* San Francisco, CA: Jossey-Bass.

Brookfield, S (1995) *Becoming a Critically Reflective Teacher.* San Francisco, CA: Jossey-Bass.

Department of Education (DfE) (2021) *Children of Critical Workers and Vulnerable Children Who Can Access Schools or Educational Settings.* [online] Available at: www.gov.uk/government/publications/coronavirus-covid-19-maintaining-educational-provision/guidance-for-schools-colleges-and-local-authorities-on-maintaining-educational-provision (accessed 20 May 2021).

Dewey, J (1933) *How We Think.* New York: DC Heath.

Dewey, J (1938) *Experience and Education.* New York: Collier Books.

Dewey, J and Bentley, A (1949) *Later Works.* Carbondale, IL: Southern Illinois University Press.

Eigege, C Y and Kennedy, P P (2021) Disruptions, Distractions, and Discoveries: Doctoral Students' Reflections on a Pandemic. *Qualitative Social Work*, 20(1–2): 618–24. Doi: 10.1177/1473325020973341.

Elfer, P and Wilson, D (2021) Talking with Feeling: Using Bion to Theorise 'Work Discussion' as a Model of Professional Reflection with Nursery Practitioners. *Pedagogy, Culture & Society* . Doi: 10.1080/14681366.2021.1895290.

Ferguson, H (2018) How Social Workers Reflect in Action and When and Why They Don't: The Possibilities and Limits to Reflective Practice in Social Work. *Social Work Education*, 37(4): 415–27.

Freire, P (1973) *Education for Critical Consciousness.* London: Sheed and Ward.

Ghaye, T, Melander-Wikman, A, Kisare, M, Chambers, P, Bergmark, U, Kostenius, C and Lillyman, S (2008) Participatory and Appreciative Action and Reflection (PAAR) – Democratizing Reflective Practices. *Reflective Practice*, 9(4): 361–97.

Gibbs, G (1988) *Learning by Doing: A Guide for Teaching and Learning Methods.* Oxford, Further education unit. Oxford Polytechnic.

Gutierrez, K and Vossoughi, S (2010) Lifting off the Ground to Return Anew: Mediated Praxis, Transformative Learning, and Social Design Experiments. *Journal of Teacher Education*, 61: 100–17. Doi: 10.1177/0022487109347877.

Hanson, K and Appleby, K (2017) *Becoming a Reflective Practitioner.* In Musgrave, J, Savin-Baden, M and Stobbs, N (eds) *Studying for Your Early Years Degree: Skills and Knowledge for Becoming an Effective Early Years Practitioner.* St Albans: Critical Publishing.

HighScope (nd) Our Approach. [online] Available at: https://highscope.org/our-practice/our-approach/ (accessed 4 May 2021).

Hochschild, A R (2003) *The Managed Heart.* London: University of California Press.

Ixer, G, 2016. The Concept of Reflection: Is It Skill Based or Values? *Social Work Education*, 35(7): 809–24.

Johnson, E (2020) Responding to Covid-19: Some Personal Reflections. *Adoption & Fostering*, 44(2): 208–11. Doi: 10.1177/0308575920934035.

Kolb, D A (1984) *Experiential Learning: Experience as the Source of Learning and Development*. New Jersey: Prentice-Hall.

Leitch, R and Day, C (2000) Action research and Reflective Practice: Towards a Holistic View. *Educational Action Research*, 8(1): 179–93.

Mezirow, J (1998) On Critical Reflection. *Adult Education Quarterly*, 48: 185–98.

Munro, E (2011) *The Munro Review of Child Protection: Final Report, A Child-Centred System*. London: The Stationery Office.

Paige-Smith, A and Craft, A (2011) Reflection and Developing a Community of Practice. In Paige-Smith, A and Craft, A (eds) *Developing Reflective Practice in the Early Years*. Berkshire: Open University Press.

Papadopoulou, M (2020) Supporting the Development of Early Years Students' Professional Identities through an Action Research Programme. *Educational Action Research*, 28(4): 686–99, doi: 10.1080/09650792.2019.1652196.

Redmond, B (2017) *Reflection in Action: Developing Reflective Practice in Health and Social Services*. Oxford: Routledge.

Reed, S M (2010) A Unitary Care Conceptual Model for Advanced Practice Nursing. *Holistic Nursing Practice*, 24(1): 23–34.

Roberts, W (2020) Reflections on Practice during a Pandemic: How Do We Continue to Ensure Effective Communication during the COVID-19 Pandemic? *Child Abuse Review*, 29: 584–8. https://doi.org/10.1002/car.2660.

Ruch, G (2007) Reflective Practice in Contemporary Child-care Social Work: The Role of Containment. *British Journal of Social Work*, 37(4): 659–80.

Schön, D A (1983) *The Reflective Practitioner*. New York: Basic Books.

Schön, D A (1988) 'From Technical Rationality to Reflection-in-Action'. In Dowie, J and Elstein, S (eds) *Professional Judgement: A Reader in Clinical Decision Making* (pp 60–76). Cambridge: Cambridge University Press.

Siegal, H (1988) *Educating Reason*. New York: Routledge.

Thompson, N and Pascal, J (2012) Developing Critically Reflective Practice. *Reflective Practice*, 13(2): 311–25.

Trodd, L and Dickerson, C (2019) 'I Enjoy Learning': Developing Early Years Practitioners' Identities as Professionals and as Professional Learners. *Professional Development in Education*, 45(3): 356–71. Doi: 10.1080/19415257.2018.1459788

Williams, A (2003) The Managed Heart: The Recognition of Emotional Labour in Public Sector Work. *Nurse Education Today*, 33: 5–7.

Part 2   Caring for yourself as a work-based learner

3 Self-care

MICHELLE MALOMO AND HAZEL RICHARDS

Self-care

- What is self-care?
- The importance of self-care
- Your self-care toolkit
- What happens when self-care is not prioritised
- Being aware of our own well-being
- Policy and practice
- Signposting and strategies

Chapter objectives ◎

This chapter considers self-care and the importance of supporting your well-being. The chapter:

- defines self-care according to current research and thinking;

- identifies the importance of self-care;

- considers what can happen when self-care is not prioritised;

- explores ways you might care for yourself as practitioners, making links to other chapters in the book;

- signposts and makes suggestions for how you might become more aware of, and support your own well-being.

Introduction

Self-care is defined by the World Health Organization (WHO) as the process of taking steps to, and engagement in activities to establish and maintain one's health (WHO, nd). The Self Care Forum (nd) adds that these actions can be taken by individuals '*themselves, on behalf of and with others in order to develop, protect, maintain and improve their health, well-being or wellness*'. Interestingly, the title of one of the references informing this chapter is '*caring for others without losing yourself*' (Neff et al, 2020) and this book, which explores areas to consider as you develop your professional identity regards self-care, in line with Neff et al (2020) as being central to this.

Theory and literature

Practitioners working in children and family support are caregivers who may also be working within cultures of self-sacrifice (Picton, 2021). Moreover, the work can be inherently demanding since it involves stressful situations and risk factors. Antonovsky explored why some people keep healthy in spite of the influence of such factors, and others don't (Antonovsky, 1987; Mittelmark et al, 2017) (see also Chapter 4). His salutogenic theory focuses on the origins of health (Antonovsky, 1979) and views health as an active, dynamic process of self-regulation meaning people can take steps to improve and maintain their own health. Self-care is an important principle in the concept of mental and physical health as it emphasises the active role individuals can play in maintaining their own well-being (Bermejo-Martins et al, 2021). It involves both agency or the ability to engage in self-care, and self-care activities carried out to keep oneself healthy (Matarese et al, 2018). This is important as practitioner self-care has been linked to increases in self-awareness, mental and physical well-being, job and life satisfaction, staff retention, personal development, effective stress management, and the ability to connect more with others and the environment (Viskovich and De George-Walker, 2019; Andrews et al, 2020).

Identifying factors that can act as improvers and maintainers of health and well-being is a necessary part of self-care (Bermejo-Martins et al, 2021). This requires us to give ourselves permission to spend time and thought on ourselves, and to show ourselves self-compassion. Strauss et al (2016) propose that compassion consists of five elements: recognising suffering, understanding the universality of human suffering, feeling for the person suffering, tolerating uncomfortable feelings and motivation to act/acting to alleviate suffering. As compassionate caregivers we are certainly used to responding to the children and families with whom we work by being non-judgemental and showing sensitivity, sympathy and empathy. However, we are perhaps less good at self-compassion.

Time to consider 💭

» What elements of your work involve self-sacrifice and how do you balance this?

» When and how do you give yourself permission to show self-care and self-compassion?

» What self-care strategies do you currently use?

The literature defines self-compassion as the ability to turn compassion inwards, to be kind to the self, and to acknowledge our humanity, imperfection and fragility (Lindström, 2014; Andrews et al, 2020). This means we must be honest with ourselves. Part of self-care therefore involves developing a positive healthy relationship with ourselves, which may mean silencing the inner critic. It also involves auditing our triggers, limits and signs and understanding and implementing behaviours and activities that can protect, maintain and improve your mental and physical health and well-being.

Time to consider 💭

» Think about your inner critic – what events or behaviours trigger it and what helps you move forward from these thoughts and the feelings they can create?

» How do you say no and limit your workload and stresses to protect yourself?

» Now identify three positive attributes that others recognise as characteristic of you. Now think of other qualities that you know you possess, but which others are less aware of.

Spotlight on new debates 🖋

How are we going to get there?

Over 2000 years ago the Greek philosopher Socrates highlighted the need to prioritise self-care. Socrates considered that although *Epimeleia heautou* – care of the self – may at first seem self-indulgent, it is in fact important that we pay attention to ourselves to be as 'good as possible' and ensure 'right conduct'. Indeed, he considered self-care to be integral to the care of others. Much more recently, the pandemic underlined the need for self-care, which has been evidenced by a plethora of publications. Andrews et al (2021) recognise that self-care can function reactively by mediating and ameliorating stress, but also, and more importantly, proactively, by identifying and implementing factors that help practitioners not merely survive, but even thrive in situations containing a multitude of challenges. These authors identify the need for their nurse participants to re-evaluate their perceptions of self-care and to 'permit' themselves time and space for it, as sometimes they had viewed it as a weakness. They also identify barriers to self-care and self-compassion, both internal (linked to identity and character) and external (linked to the environment, organisational expectations and practice – see section on policy and practice in settings below).

Identifying internal barriers to self-care and self-compassion is part of being honest and being able to make a realistic evaluation of our attitudes, understandings, strengths and challenges. It is therefore closely linked to our self-awareness and developing identities. Identifying internal barriers to self-care and self-compassion may also require us to re-evaluate their role – not as coping strategies resorted to only when we are overwhelmed, but as a part of our practitioner toolkits. Toolkits can be viewed either as a set of tools, kept in one place and used for a particular purpose or as '*a personal set of resources, abilities, or skills*' (Lexico, nd). Whichever definition you apply, a toolkit conveys the idea of a range of tools that can be used in various combinations, and which are within reach because they are located in a known place. Relating this to self-care, this section now uses current research to explore some 'tools' that you might find helpful to have in your own personal toolkit.

A range of 'tools' exist that we have linked to research. Hasson (2020) and Viskovitch and De George-Walker (2019) identify the central role of self-knowledge to self-care. This is like the measuring tape, where we measure and get to know our reach but also our limits. Andrews et al (2021) suggest that we need to feel safe and secure in ourselves and our workplace to be self-caring and self-compassionate. This is like the spirit level that reveals how level or centred our base is. Working through the pandemic required keyworkers to balance stresses at both work and home. Elliot et al's (2021) study recognised the need for genuine kindness and provision of support for staff. This is like the screw clamp that helps hold things together. The importance of building healthy lifestyles to support our physical and psychological well-being (Emery, 2020; Neff et al, 2020) could be likened to several different tools. In contrast, keeping up the appearance of coping while maintaining patient care, despite inadequate time and care to deal with our own individual emotional responses (Mills et al, 2020; Galiana et al, 2021), could be conceptualised as the paint and brush, though this is only a temporary solution in that without addressing the underlying issue, cracks and peeling will occur in time.

Time to consider 💭

Self-care involves identifying what does and doesn't work for you, which may be different for you when life is just jogging along to when life is more difficult and challenging. This is similar to using different combinations of tools for different jobs.

» Can you identify which of the described self-care 'tools' you use and the different times or situations you might employ these in?

What can happen when self-care is not prioritised?

Work supporting children and families involves high levels of care and there can be a heightened risk of practitioner's own well-being being adversely affected by the sometimes intense demands of the job (Neff et al, 2020). The pandemic increased safeguarding issues. It also challenged the mental health of many children and families (Romanou et al, 2020). The children and families workforce were recognised as key workers, and most experienced extra stress and upset in the course of their work as a result of these and other issues (Mills et al, 2020; Nelinger et al, 2021; Bermejo-Martins et al, 2021; Elliot et al, 2021).

Proactive self-care has been shown to reduce adverse effects such as levels of compassion fatigue, burnout and stress (Andrews et al, 2020). However, for many of us, with so much to do and think about, self-care can easily fall by the wayside (Hasson, 2020). This is serious. Self-care is considered to be an ethical imperative in certain fields such as psychology, since practising without adequate self-care strategies may, at best, mean less effective practice, or at worst, mean practitioners are working while psychologically impaired and potentially impacting service user outcomes and well-being (Viskovich and De George-Walker, 2019). It is also serious because inadequate practitioner self-care can contribute to damaging consequences for the individual such as distress, the loss of job satisfaction, poor psychological health and self-medicating behaviours.

Moving forward, it is therefore perhaps more important than ever to monitor and be aware of any changes in your behaviour that may suggest your current self-care is not adequately maintaining your health and well-being (Hasson, 2020). Differences in your sleep patterns and feeling tired or sluggish can indicate that you need to prioritise self-care. Feelings of emptiness, disconnection and loneliness, or struggling to feel optimistic and locate a sense of purpose can be other signs (Schechter et al, 2020). However, while authors such as Hasson (2020) provide a comprehensive list of signs and symptoms to look out for, we acknowledge we are not experts in physical and psychological distress ourselves. The chapter therefore aims to be solutions focused, so in line with salutogenesis is concerned with proactive self-care. This is because promoting a healthy lifestyle, such as a healthy diet, physical activity or sleep (Bermejo-Martins et al, 2021), and psychological resources such as emotional intelligence (EI), mindfulness and reflection skills, can serve as important assets to decrease the negative effects of stress while increasing the health, well-being and resilience of practitioners. The following sections of this chapter therefore focus on external factors (policy and practice in settings) and internal factors (solutions and strategies as well as resources) that you might consider as you develop your self-care toolkit.

Policy and practice in settings: an emphasis on mental health and well-being

Valuing self-care should not be viewed as an indulgence, rather it should be an essential component of professionalism (Barnett and Cooper, 2009). This thought is central to this book. However, regarding self-care as essential is an aspirational mindset for all who work within the children and family sector – not only for you but also for the children and families that you work with and we know that for some practitioners in the field this component of professionalism is lacking. So, how can this aspiration become a strategy that has meaningful expression within workplaces?

Cleary et al (2020, p 4) state that the implementation of self-care and mutual care strategies within the workplace enhances the mental health and professional well-being of practitioners. They also go further in suggesting that

> Leaders and teams can foster innovative well-being opportunities to promote healthy workplace knowledge, attitudes and behaviours and build resilient and humane workplace cultures.

This thinking offers some potentially helpful solutions and will help you to unpack and discover solutions around self-care that can be implemented within the workplace.

Creating a self-care culture

First, workplaces that have a culture that promotes not only self-care but also mutual-care strategies will enhance the mental health and well-being of those within the setting. Mutual care is a reciprocal and collaborative process that involves co-production of solutions and joint or team implementation of support. This means creating a culture and workplace that values not only self-care initiatives but that also ensures self-care becomes fundamental to the setting's values. This may mean creating and developing both policy and practice that is personally meaningful to your workplace team. Consider the following question to support you in thinking about such possible solutions.

Critical questions ⑦

» If you could work in an environment that valued self-care and mutual care what characteristics or practice might you be able to see?

Often the media highlights Mental Health Week and we may celebrate this by having a focus on self-care within the workplace. This is a positive start but often can feel tokenistic in creating a meaningful self-care and mutual care culture. However, such events can give you an insight into strategies that might be more sustainable in your workplaces. Consider the next questions.

» Has this occurred in your workplace? How did initiatives on this day make you feel?

» How might this help in thinking about longer term sustainable self-care and mutual care practice? Note down your thoughts and ideas.

Second, the responsibility for developing this culture falls not only to those that lead but also to the wider team. This is because developing a self-care culture within a workplace requires knowledge of self-care which in turn fosters attitudes that promote well-being. What also resonates here is a culture where there is mutual respect and a spirit of kindness that supports practice development. Allies (2021) states that having a culture where mental health is discussed openly helps to normalise conversation around well-being. Once this happens it can have a significant impact in culture change. While initially this will take courage and bravery, the increasing challenges brought by the pandemic means the need to recognise and discuss those challenges is increasingly acknowledged and accepted.

Allies (2021) also suggests that leaders need to model positive self-care by having an awareness of and managing their own self-care. This may not always be seen in practice, and we can have an expectation that any culture change must be developed through the example of setting leaders. Where this is not the case, cultures can be created when team members take the lead. Burns (1978) suggests that the Transformational Leadership can inspire the team to change practice to achieve positive and desired outcomes and to bring about good for the whole team. This model of leadership may not be led by the actual leader or manager within the setting so could bring about the change that is needed for the team. Indeed, that person could be you.

How can I create a culture of self-care within my setting?

The following points are suggested to open discussion around developing and enhancing cultures of self-care, in particular as an agenda for a team meeting.

- Ask for self-care to be on the next team meeting agenda.

  Ask the team for suggestions for how the setting could create a sustainable self-care culture that is part of the whole year – not just as part of mental health awareness week. Allies (2021, p 130) suggests that these can be small things that make a big difference, for example, working together to give everyone their birthday as a day off. Other ideas could be arranging well-being enhancing days which could include walks in the countryside with a pub lunch, exercising together, spa days or just exploring books or a hobby together. Collect ideas that are meaningful to your team so that you can create a well-being calendar for the team.

- Within coaching and supervision (see Chapter 9), ask for self-care to be a regular discussion item within your mentee or supervision sessions.

  To ensure this practice is developed and becomes part of the culture of the setting, suggest that a smaller working party from within the team liaises to develop a self-care policy within staff guidance for promoting a self-care culture for all in the setting – including staff, children and their families.

  You might also like to share resources from Mental Health First Aid England (2021) with your team – these support the creation of a culture of self-care within the workplace.

  In summary, Allies (2021, p 21) suggests that talking '*openly about any mental health and well-being problems*' is at the heart of creating a culture of self-care. This may involve you being at the heart of this discussion and seeking solutions within your workplace.

Signposting, solutions and strategies

So far this chapter has explored theories highlighting the importance of self-care, highlighted the importance of self-care within society, and offered suggestions as to how you might start a discussion around creating and co-constructing a culture of self-care within your workplace. As authors of this chapter, we do not claim to be experts in this area but what we do have is a passion to promote self-care as a solution to the potential for burnout we see within the sector. The pandemic has affected each one of us in some way and The Mental Health Foundation (2020, p 3) suggests the effects will be felt for some time *'but there is also cause for hope. While there is no vaccine for mental distress, much can be done to prevent mental health problems; well evidenced solutions are at hand'*. Therefore, this section of the chapter will offer a range of tools and suggestions of possible solutions by highlighting strategies developed by experts within the field.

Certainly, reading and researching for this chapter has uncovered numerous helpful and supportive signposts although it is evident that to be able to really care for ourselves we need to invest time with intention. Gobin (2019, p 5) offers a poignant insight here, stating that '*self-care is about taking a serious look in the mirror and making changes that will give your life more balance, meaning, purpose and fulfilment'*. Gobin (2019) suggests that to be able to understand self-care we need to really understand ourselves and our needs before we begin to seek solutions. This may not be easy as many of us have been conditioned to think that time thinking about self is selfish or self-indulgent. This perspective is not true and is a misconception that can prevent engagement with a self-care plan. Therefore, in line with this book's focus on developing your professional identity, take a moment to reflect on you and your own self-care needs before the chapter moves on to seeking your own personalised solutions.

Time to consider ☁

» Think of a place where you can be alone with yourself. This may be walking in the outdoors or sitting on your favourite chair. But it could also mean locking yourself in the bathroom if that is the only place where you can be alone!

» Once in your 'place' just take a few deep breaths in and out. It is helpful to place your feet firmly on the floor just to ground yourself. This might seem a luxury as far as time is concerned. It is not.

» You may find it helpful to have a notepad (which could become your self-care journal). Just note here the thoughts that are passing through your head – this will help declutter your mind before we move on to consider your individual self-care needs.

» Take a moment – what thoughts have you jotted down? Do these give any insights into areas of self-care that you may need to focus upon?

> » Now think about the areas of your self-care that you think you may need to focus upon. Please don't worry if you are unsure about these since the next part of this chapter will support you.

Developing a meaningful and achievable self-care plan

Good self-care needs to be developed as a habit. For example, cleaning our teeth, limiting sugary drinks, flossing and regular dental check-ups with a dentist are all good habits and necessary for good oral healthcare. In the same way, we need to have a shift in our mindset to develop a self-care plan and behaviours that make self-care, and its maintenance, part of our day-to-day routine. Although when starting out these may seem a luxury, such habits are an essential component of good mental health.

To start with, it is helpful to undertake an audit of your approaches to self-care and use this information to help you develop your personalised self-care plan. An excellent resource to support this initial assessment has been developed by the NHS (2021). As part of its Better Health resources, it has developed Every Mind Matters (please see the link in the table below). You can access an online survey on Every Mind Matters that considers all aspects of your mental health. After this is completed, you will be sent an overview of a personal plan that will support you, including resources to help your focus when developing your self-care plan.

Another useful resource has been developed by Mental Health First Aid England (2021). This resource is part of their 'My Whole Self' resources and is called the 'Whole Self MOT'. This resource provides a good start and supports the development of a self-care plan. It uses a series of questions and would work well alongside a self-care journal. It can also be used as a check-in resource as an on-going evaluation of your well-being. The link to access this resource can be found in Table 3.1.

Finally, if you prefer not to access online sources then Gobin's (2019) book *The Self-care Prescription* is very helpful. This resource is a self-care course wrapped up in a book. Each chapter supports you in making plans to develop your well-being. This is just a different way you can develop a workable self-care plan.

Whichever resource you use to help create your self-care plan, it is important that you focus on the different aspects of maintaining healthy well-being through focusing on each of these. To support your thinking, we have envisioned self-care as being like a hub with spokes (see Figure 3.1), each of which need to be maintained for positive self-care.

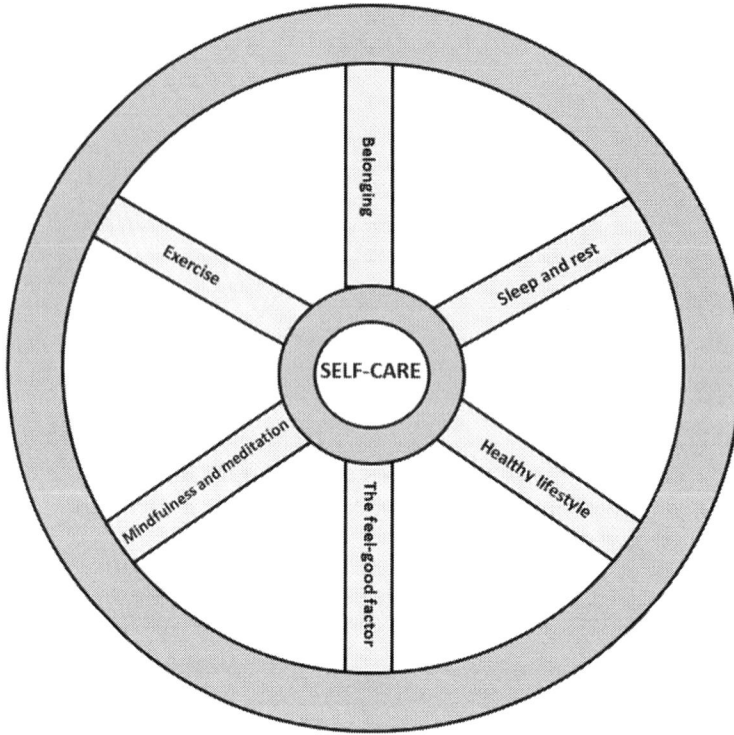

Figure 3.1 *The well-being wheel. Adapted from NHS (2021) and Gobin (2019)*

The spokes in our well-being wheel are made up of the following areas: exercise; mindfulness and meditation; the feel-good factor; healthy lifestyle; sleep and rest; and belonging. These spokes of well-being summarise best practice and resources that have been developed by experts. In Table 3.1 the spokes are used to group resources that might help you to develop and sustain your self-care plans. The intention is that you use these resources to develop a personally meaningful and sustainable approach to your own self-care.

Table 3.1 *Self-care and well-being resources*

Overview of resource	How can I access?
Self-care plan development resources	
Get Your Mind Plan is part of the NHS resources Every Mind Matters resources and supports you through a short survey to develop a mind plan. You will be sent the plan via email, and you will receive regular email check-ins.	Available at: www.nhs.uk/every-mind-matters/mental-well-being-tips/your-mind-plan-quiz/
The My Whole Self MOT resource is part of the Mental Health First Aid England My Whole Self resources and supports you in developing a regular and developmental self-care check-in.	Available at: https://mhfaengland.org/my-whole-self/resources/

Table 3.1 (*Cont.*)

Overview of resource	How can I access?
The Self-care Prescription is a book that takes you on a journey of discovery that examines what you might need for your personalised self-care prescription.	Gobins, R L (2018) *The Self-care Prescription*. Emeryville, CA: Althea Press.

Exercise

You may have a favoured exercise method and it is important that you try to achieve the recommended 150 minutes per week. But if you are looking for some inspiration the sources in this section may help.

The Couch-to-5k is an NHS resource and is one way in which you can improve the amount of time you exercise.	Available at: www.nhs.uk/live-well/exercise/couch-to-5k-week-by-week/
The NHS has a fitness studio where you can access a variety of online exercise videos.	Available at: www.nhs.uk/conditions/nhs-fitness-studio/
The NHS also recommends pages that can support you to explore an exercise mode that motivates you. This page covers a variety of exercise and allows you to explore a variety of exercises to get inspired.	Available at: www.thisgirlcan.co.uk/activities/
Finally, the power of walking is explored in the following NHS resource – even just ten minutes a day can make a difference.	Available at: www.nhs.uk/live-well/exercise/walking-for-health/

Mindfulness and meditation

Headspace meditation is a helpful website with an accompanying downloadable app, developed by Andy Puddicombe, a meditation and mindfulness expert.	Available at: www.headspace.com/meditation and www.headspace.com/mindfulness
NHS Mindfulness links to a variety of helpful sources that can support you with developing the practice of mindfulness, including links to short videos.	Available at: www.nhs.uk/mental-health/self-help/tips-and-support/mindfulness/
Mindfulness for Students is a book that considers the value of mindfulness when studying. Written by Stella Cottrell, who is considered a study skills guru, students who have used this have found it really helpful.	Cottrell, S (2018) *Mindfulness for Students*. London: Palgrave

→

Table 3.1 (*Cont.*)

Overview of resource	How can I access?
The feel-good factor	
This section involves developing social situations which could involve meeting with friends or even taking up a new hobby. Essential to this solution is having fun and enjoyment.	
The Self-care Prescription book has some very helpful chapters. Research a hobby that you would like to take up. How might you develop this?	Gobins, R L (2018) *The Self-care Prescription*. Specifically: Chapter 2 Friends, Family and Fun – Social Self-care Chapter 7 Be Your Own Best Friend – Emotional Self-care
Healthy lifestyle	
This section focuses on eating well.	
The NHS provides researched and accepted approaches to healthy eating. This is a good starting place for improving your approach to food and nutrition and its important place in your self-care.	Available at: www.nhs.uk/live-well/eat-well/eight-tips-for-healthy-eating/
The NHS has also produced the Eat Well pages. These support you in looking at how and what you eat and how this can promote good self-care.	Available at: www.nhs.uk/live-well/eat-well/the-eatwell-guide/
Sleep and rest	
The Rethinking Rest resource developed by the Mental Health Organisation is designed for education settings but is useful to anyone who wishes to explore what rest means to you personally.	Available at: www.mentalhealth.org.uk/sites/default/files/ENGLISH.%20Rethinking%20Rest.pdf
'How sleep and green space can help your mental health' is a podcast developed by The Mental Health Foundation and research scientist Julie Dunn (University of Liverpool) exploring that power of outdoor spaces and their connection with sleep.	Available at: www.mentalhealth.org.uk/podcasts-and-videos/how-sleep-and-green-space-can-help-your-mental-health
Mind has developed a helpful webpage with suggestions as to how you might improve sleep patterns.	Available at: www.mind.org.uk/information-support/types-of-mental-health-problems/sleep-problems/tips-to-improve-your-sleep/

Table 3.1 (*Cont.*)

Overview of resource	How can I access?
Belonging	
The survey in the NHS, Every Mind Matters resources may highlight the importance of thinking about where you belong, and suggests that one way to address this is volunteering, since giving to others and having a sense of belonging can be very helpful in supporting you to maintain your well-being.	Available at: https://volunteeringmatters.org.uk/

In presenting the resources above we hope that you have been able to develop your own well-being tool kit. There is a wealth of support and solutions. We hope the information in the table supports you also in taking that step by step plan to understanding your own needs but also recognise that it is a process that will require some time, but you can take this step by step. These resources are all accessible at the time of writing and many are free and it is hoped that they are therefore accessible and open to all.

Chapter summary 📖

This chapter has explored the need for and value of self-care. It has identified key areas to consider and has signposted you to a range of potential solutions and strategies that will support you in developing a self-care plan, while leaving you as an individual reader to make the decision about what works for you.

Further reading 📚

Allies, S (2020) *Supporting Teacher Well-being: A Practical Guide for Primary Teachers and School Leaders*. Oxford: Routledge.

- This is a very readable book that supports anyone within the children and families' sector. Lots of very helpful and practical suggestions.

Gobin, L (2019) *The Self care Prescription: Powerful Solutions to Manage Stress, Reduce Anxiety and Increase Well-being*. Emeryville, CA: Althea Press.

- This is an excellent resource if you prefer a text rather than a website. It takes you through developing a self-care plan, chapter by chapter.

Zahariades, D (2020) *The Mental Toughness Handbook*. Art of Productivity.

- This book is full of practical ideas that develop a mental toughness through reflective ideas.

References ≋

Allies, S (2020) *Supporting Teacher Well-being: A Practical Guide for Primary Teachers and School Leaders*. Oxford: Routledge.

Andrews, H, Tierney, S and Seers K (2020) Needing Permission: The Experience of Self-care and Self-compassion in Nursing: A Constructivist Grounder Theory Study. *International Journal of Nursing Studies*, 101: 103436.

Antonovsky, A (1979) *Health, Stress and Coping: New Perspectives on Mental and Physical Well-being*. San Francisco: Josef Bass.

Antonovsky, A (1987) *Unravelling the Mystery of Health; How People Manage Stress and Stay Well*. San-Francisco: Jossey-Bass.

Barnett, J E and Cooper, N (2009) Creating a Culture of Self-care. *Clinical Psychology: Science and Practice*, 16(1): 16–20.

Bermejo-Martins, E, Luis, E O, Fernandez-Berrocal, P, Martínez, M and Sarrionandia, A (2021) The Role of Emotional Intelligence and Self-care in the Stress Perception during COVID-19 Outbreak: An Intercultural Moderated Mediation Analysis. *Personality and Individual Differences*, 177: 110679.

Cleary, M, Schafer, C, McLean, L and Visentin, D C (2020) Mental Health and Well-being in the Health Workplace. *Issues in Mental Health Nursing*, 41(2): 172–5. Doi: 10.1080/01612840.2019.1701937.

Cottrell, S (2018) *Mindfulness for Students*. London: Palgrave.

Elliot, R, Crowe, L, Abbenbroek, B, Grattam, S and Hammond, N (2021) Critical Care Health Professionals' Self-reported Needs for Well-being during the COVID-19 Pandemic: A Thematic Analysis of Survey Responses. *Australian Critical Care*, https://doi.org/10.1016/j.aucc.2021.08.007

Emery, S (2020) The Importance of Self-care for Improving Student Nurse Well-being. *British Journal of Nursing*, 29(14): 830.

Galiana, L, Sanso, N, Munoz-Martinez, I, Vidal-Blanco, G, Oliver, A and Larkin, P (2021) Palliative Care Professional's Inner Life: Exploring the Mediating Role of Self-compassion in the Prediction of Compassion Satisfaction, Compassion Fatigue, Burnout and Well-being. *Journal of Pain and Symptom Management*, 63(1): 112–23.

Gobin, L (2019) *The Self-Care Prescription: Powerful Solutions to Manage Stress, Reduce Anxiety and Increase Well-being*. Emeryville, CA: Althea Press.

Hasson, G (2020) *The Self-care Handbook: Connect with Yourself and Boost Your Well-being*. Edina, MN: Capstone.

Lexico (nd). 'Toolkit' Definition. [online] Available at: www.lexico.com/definition/toolkit (accessed 20 January 2022).

Lindström, S (2014) *Self-compassion: I Don't Have to Feel Better than Others to Feel Good about Myself*. Marston Gate: Amazon.

Matarese, M, Lommi, M, De Marinis, M G and Riegel, B (2018) A Systematic Review and Integration of Concept Analyses of Self-care and Related Concepts. *Journal of Nursing Scholarship*, 50(3): 296–305.

Mental Health First Aid England (2021) My Whole Self Free Resources. [online] Available at: https://mhfaengland.org/my-whole-self/resources/ (accessed 20 January 2022).

Mills, J, Ramachenderan, J, Chapman, M, Greenland, R and Agar, M (2020) Prioritising Workforce Well-being and Resilience: What COVID-19 Is Reminding Us about Self-care and Staff Support. *Palliative Medicine*, 34(9): 1137–9.

Mittelmark, M B, Bull, T and Bowman, L (2017) Emerging Ideas Relevant to the Salutogenic Model of Health. In Mittelmark, M, Sagy, S, Eriksoon, M, Bauer, G, Pelikan, J, Lindström, B and Espnes, G (eds) *The Handbook of Salutogenesis*. Cham: Springer.

Neff, K D, Knox, M C, Long, P and Gregory, K (2020) Caring for Others Without Losing Yourself: An Adaptation of the Mindful Self-compassion Program for Healthcare Communities. *Journal of Clinical Psychology*, 76(9): 1543–62.

Nelinger, A, Album, J, Haynes, A and Rosan, C (2021) *Their Challenges Are Our Challenges: A Summary Report of the Experiences Facing Nursery Workers in the UK in 2020*. Anna Freud National Centre for Children and Families. [online] Available at: www.annafreud.org/media/13013/their-challenges-are-our-challenges-survey-report.pdf (accessed 3 November 2021).

Picton, A (2021) Work-Life Balance in Medical Students: Self-care in a Culture of Self-sacrifice. *BMC Medical Education*, 21(8): 1–12.

Romanou, E and Belton, E (2020) *Isolated and Struggling: Social Isolation and the Risk of Child Maltreatment, in Lockdown and Beyond*. NSPCC Learning, https://learning.nspcc.org.uk/media/2246/isolated-and-struggling-social-isolation-risk-childmaltreatment-lockdown-and-beyond.pdf (accessed 20 January 2022).

Self Care Forum (nd) Helping People Take Care of Themselves. [online] Available at: www.self-careforum.org (accessed 3 November 2021).

Shechter, A, Diaz, F, Moise, N, Anstey, D E, Ye, S, Agarwal, S, Birk, J L, Brodie, D, Cannone, D E, Chang, B and Claassen, J (2020) Psychological Distress, Coping Behaviors, and Preferences for Support among New York Healthcare Workers during the COVID-19 Pandemic. *General Hospital Psychiatry*, 66: 1–8.

Strauss, C, Taylor, B L, Gu, J, Kuyken, W, Baer, R, Jones, F and Kate Cavanagh, K (2016) What Is Compassion and How Can We Measure It? A Review of Definitions and Measures. *Clinical Psychology Review*, 47: 15–27.

Viskovitch, S and De George-Walker, L (2019) An Investigation of Self-care Constructs in Undergraduate Psychology Students: Self-compassion, Mindfulness, Self-awareness and Integrated Self-knowledge. *International Journal of Educational Research*, 95: 109–17.

World Health Organization (nd) Self-care Interventions for Health. [online] Available at: www.who.int/health-topics/self-care (accessed 3 November 2021).

4 Resilience

MICHELLE MALOMO

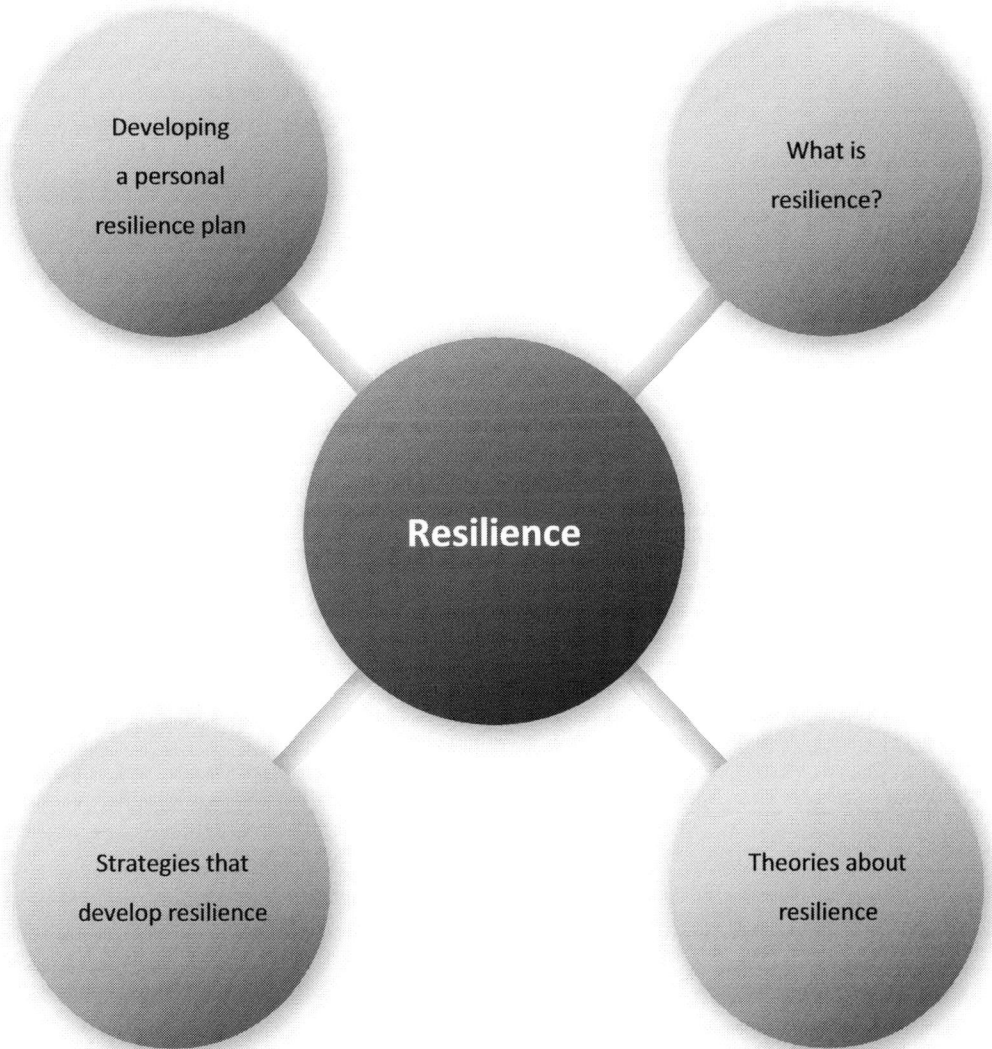

(They) stood in the storm and when the wind did not blow (them) away, they adjusted their sails.

Elizabeth Edwards (2009)

Chapter objectives ◎

The chapter:

* attempts to define resilience;

* considers theory and thinking concerning resilience both personally and in the workplace;

* explores strategies that develop resilience;

* supports you to develop a personal resilience plan.

Introduction

Writing this chapter has extended my own knowledge as well as evoking a personal discovery of how resilience has sustained me throughout my own professional practice.

Reflection is a critical component in understanding the value of resilience. This is because gaining a meaningful understanding of resilience will involve returning to life events, examining responses, and deciding how you might develop your resilient spirit both personally, and as you develop your professional identity.

What is resilience?

It is important to acknowledge the fascinating and elusive nature of resilience at the start of this chapter. This is because students often seek definitive answers when exploring concepts. However, concepts can be 'slippery' and may need to be experienced to be fully understood. Also, resilience has been defined in several ways (King et al, 2016) so arriving at a definitive definition is challenging. Neenan (2018, p 4) suggests that,

> *Resilience is an intriguing yet elusive concept: intriguing because it can provide some sort of answer as to why one person crumbles in the face of tough times while another gains strength from them, but elusive in that the concept resists a definitive definition.*

When attempting to define resilience, it is important that you hold the thoughts explored lightly, and through the reflective tasks within this chapter you develop a definition of resilience that is personally meaningful. Below we will start to consider some of the possible definitions.

Fletcher and Sarkar (2013) suggest that adversity proceeds resilience and contributes to adaptations that positively build resilience. Other definitions suggest that resilience is the ability to bounce back from adversity (Grant and Kinman, 2015; Rajan-Rankin, 2014). However, bouncing back from adversity is often a challenging process that takes time, and this phrase fails to acknowledge that the process can include suffering and struggle (Walsh, 2016). Neenan (2018) helpfully suggests that although bouncing back can make you a stronger, better person, this is not the reality for everyone. He suggests that 'bouncing back' implies that we return to a pre-adversity state or place and this is just not possible. Mu (2021) argues that it is important not to accept the notion that resilience is a tool for absorption, for adapting and then just returning to the original place that we inhabited before we experienced the adversity. Instead we may need to challenge the process that led us to this place. Indeed, it appears that many of us do not bounce back. Having considered this, we will all experience challenge or adversity. During these times it may just feel as if we take small steps through the experience, and it is our resilient spirit that supports us in just facing the situation day by day. Then at some point we will be able to make progress in our outlook and move beyond the processing of the experience. This feels like we bounce forward into a new space in our thinking and possibly our practice. While working with children and their families you will pass through experiences that will potentially challenge you and which will require you to manage your responses.

In defining resilience, it is important then to recognise that our responses to adversity are unique and shaped by our past experiences, personality and the environment that we experience the challenges within. Tugade and Fredrickson (2004, p 1) highlight that 'resilient individuals have optimistic, zestful, and energetic approaches to life, are curious and open to new experiences, and are characterized by high positive emotionality'. This definition suggests that resilience is linked to personality traits but also offers some suggestion as to how we might achieve and further develop a resilient nature. The works of Fredrickson, including some of the strategies that she suggests might help us to develop traits that support resilience, are considered in more depth later in the chapter.

Resilience can also be seen from a psychological perspective. Barthélemy et al (2020, p 281) suggest that resilience is multidimensional and involves the ability to adapt positively to life conditions. This definition also suggests resilience is dynamic, involves taking time to adapt and supports the individual to 'face difficulties by observing an initial balance or bouncing back as an opportunity for growth'. Seeing resilience in this manner suggests it is a concept or trait that can grow in the individual. This aligns with the thinking within this book, that is, that professional identity is ever developing.

Time to consider ☁

» If you were to define resilience what would be your first thoughts?

» Having worked through some of the thoughts expressed by others in the literature, how has your understanding developed?

» Reflecting upon the responses you have made to the above questions – how would you now define resilience?

Understanding how the brain affects resilience

In recent years I have become more aware that understanding how the brain works can inform our practice with children and their families. When considering how resilience is defined it appears that the neurobiological response we have to adversity and stress affects our personal levels of resilience and in turn, how we develop the attributes of resilience. Barthélemy et al (2020, p 281) suggest that understanding neuroscience can support our understanding as to why we respond differently to adversity. Having some knowledge of this is also helpful when defining resilience as it appears that resilience is seen as a state of mind. Knowing and understanding some basic neuroscience of how the brain and body respond to adversity and stress will support you in understanding your individual responses and which tools and strategies may be best to support you in becoming more resilient.

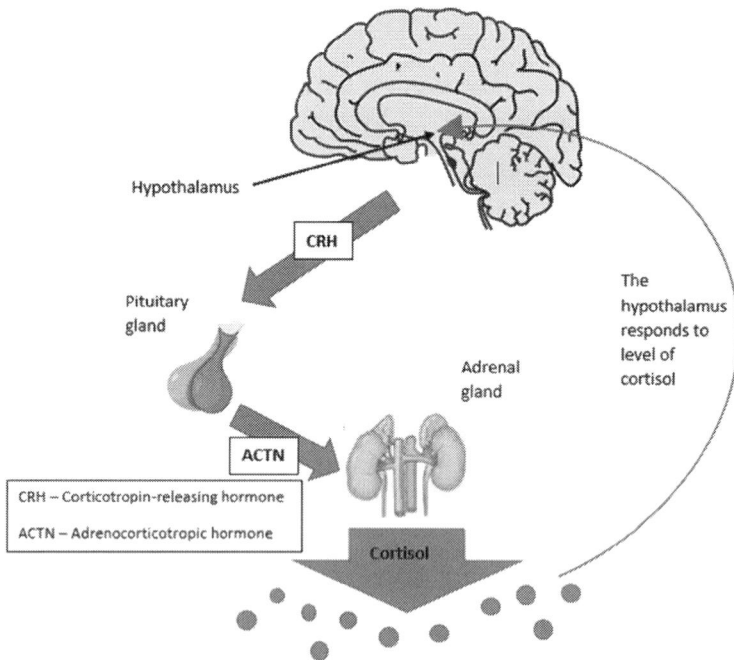

Figure 4.1 *The stress response system*

Understanding our brain responses to stress is supported by a basic understanding of the hypothalamic pituitary adrenal (HPA) axis. Figure 4.1 gives a visual representation of the HPA axis. The HPA axis describes the interaction between the hypothalamus, pituitary gland and adrenal glands. When experiencing stressful situations, the hypothalamus triggers the release of corticotropin-releasing hormone into the pituitary gland. The pituitary glands then release adrenocorticotropic hormone into the adrenal gland. The adrenal glands then produce cortisol, and once cortisol is produced the hypothalamus responds. The hypothalamus is responsible for controlling many of the body's responses including body temperature, thirst, appetite and weight control, emotions, sleep cycles and even blood pressure and heart rate. This list highlights that our body and brain produce physical responses when we experience extreme stress. Indeed, our body is wired with an alarm system when we experience adversity. Knowing this is helpful. Controlling these responses and rewiring our bodies alarm system may partially explain individual capacity to show resilience. Knowledge can support you in understanding strategies and tools that will support you in developing our personal levels of resilience.

Time to consider 💭

» Having explored the HPA axis, can you think of a time either personally or within your working life where you experienced a heightened level of stress?

» How did you feel your body responded to this? It may be helpful to consider the list of responses above.

» Do you feel that when you feel stressed you adopt a particular mindset? Can you describe the feelings that you have experienced?

» How do you feel you might be able to become resilient when facing adversity? What approaches are available, and how can you develop these further?

Resilience both personally and in the workplace

King et al (2015) suggest that we all need to show resilience within child and family work given that adversity will inevitably be experienced by a team working together at some point. Showing resilience in work is connected to our personal ability to develop it, and '*there is growing evidence that resilience can be developed through the use of cognitive transformation and personal growth training*' (King et al 2015, p 783). This highlights that having a positive mindset can have an impact, though work-based cultures will influence your responses.

Neenan (2018) suggests that one of the secrets of developing a resilient spirit within the workplace is to find an '*inner stability*'. Resilience developed in this manner will prevent you feeling overtly overwhelmed or stressed. Kinman et al (2020) highlight that for many social workers the job brings stress and although there is a responsibility on the organisation, personal emotional resilience also needs to be developed to be able to cope with the demands of the profession. This suggests that some of the responsibility for being resilient in the workplace is yours, which means that you have effective strategies for managing your responses in challenging situations. However, this does not excuse either workplace employers or government social policy from promoting and supporting the well-being of those employed within the sector, since they too have responsibility for ensuring organisational cultures value the well-being of employees.

This is often challenging. The recent and continuing Covid-19 pandemic has put unbelievable stress on the sector. For example, despite the childcare sector being essential in supporting and releasing keyworkers for work, funding was cut, placing private sector childcare businesses at the brink of survival (Blanden et al, 2020). This placed practitioners at risk of losing their jobs in addition to already risking their own health and well-being. Having spoken to practitioners and students who were working at the coalface during this time, it seemed that they remained resilient by placing trust in each other and pulling together. Students working in the sector expressed frustrations and fears of working in the pandemic. They also recognised that talking to other practitioners about how they felt helped. The ability to have a sense of humour lightened the load as well. They also said that having family there to support them at the end of the day was helpful. Allies (2021) suggests that it is important to have an awareness that everyone within a workplace will have varying sensitivity to stress and stressful situations. She stresses that it is important to develop a culture where peers check in with each other, as this lessens the isolation that can be felt in stressful circumstances and creates a culture of trust where problems can be discussed.

Working with children and their families means that no two days are the same. The work, as discussed in Chapter 5, requires an empathetic approach and this requires energy. Rose and Palatini (2020) suggest that it is similarly important to develop a set of emotional boundaries alongside reflective self-care management since these are also required to sustain resilience. They highlight, however, that often these emotional boundaries are elusive. Policies within the workplace could support practitioners for this to be achieved (see Chapter 3).

Critical questions ⑦

Work-based policies that support resilience

»   Thinking about working in practice, which policies (if any) are in place to support your well-being?

»   What review or development of these policies could support you in maintaining your well-being and resilience within the workplace?

»   Where you have policies that outline partnerships and multi-agency working, what procedures are in place to support emotional boundaries within this work?

»   How are policies reviewed within your workplace and how can you contribute to this process?

Exploring strategies that develop resilience

Having explored explanations of what resilience might be, this section examines two theories that may be helpful when developing resilience. These will support you in thinking about how you might then develop your own personalised resilience tool kit.

The Resilience Framework

The Resilience Framework was originally developed to support children and young people to become resilient and to recognise resilient traits they were already displaying (Hart, Blincow and Thomas, 2007). This was later adapted into a framework for adults which can be seen in Figure 4.2. The Resilience Framework has five key elements that help develop a resilient approach or strategy. These are basics, belonging, learning, coping and core self.

	BASICS	BELONGING	LEARNING	COPING	CORE SELF
SPECIFIC APPROACHES	Good enough housing	Find somewhere for the child/YP to belong	Make school/college life work as well as possible	Understanding boundaries and keeping within them	Instil a sense of hope
		Help child/YP understand their place in the world		Being brave	
	Enough money to live	Tap into good influences	Engage mentors for children/YP		Support the child/YP to understand other people's feelings
	Being safe	Keep relationships going		Solving problems	
	Access & transport	The more healthy relationships the better	Map out career or life plan	Putting on rose-tinted glasses	Help the child/YP to know her/himself
		Take what you can from relationships where there is some hope		Fostering their interests	
	Healthy diet	Get together people the child/YP can count on	Help the child/YP to organise her/himself	Calming down & self-soothing	Help the child/YP take responsibility for her/himself
		Responsibilities & obligations			
	Exercise and fresh air	Focus on good times and places	Highlight achievements	Remember tomorrow is another day	Foster their talents
	Enough sleep	Make sense of where child/YP has come from		Lean on others when necessary	
	Play & leisure	Predict a good experience of someone or something new	Develop life skills		There are tried and tested treatments for specific problems, use them
	Being free from prejudice & discrimination	Make friends and mix with other children/YPs		Have a laugh	
	NOBLE TRUTHS				
	ACCEPTING	CONSERVING	COMMITMENT		ENLISTING

Figure 4.2 Resilience framework (adults) – copyright Hart, Blincow and Cameron (2007) (adapted from original) www.boingboing.org.uk

Basics

Hart, Blincow and Cameron (2007) suggest that having the basics of life has been overlooked in much of the writings on resilience theory and suggest that having these in place is a good starting point. The basic element of the framework is concerned with the physical and psychological needs that need to be in place if we are to function effectively. For example, if you aren't sleeping well it will create challenges for your work and resilience. They suggest that if you are struggling to see positives as you navigate your way through adversity, assessing your basics of life can help identify what you do have in place to support you. Acknowledging this can help you reframe your own thinking.

Belonging

The belonging element highlights the importance of relationships and how using relationships to good effect can support us in becoming resilient. The belonging element also involves developing the ability to recognise the influences of good and bad relationships and how these can either support or cause disturbances to your own sense of resilience. When exploring the framework this element may offer a real challenge to your own thinking as it is not easy being honest about the impact certain relationships, and belonging, may be having on your resilient spirit.

Learning

When looking at the framework it is interesting that embracing learning is seen as a key element. Many of the themes reflected within this element are also reflected within this book. Being able to embrace the opportunities to learn from experiences, people and the right environment can support us in developing a resilient spirit. It is also worth recognising that you can learn when the reverse happens too – experiences that you might perceive as failures are opportunities to learn. This element resonated with my own professional identity journey, and I can see how struggling and sometimes failing have empowered me to keep going.

Coping

The next two elements within the framework need to be seen in parallel. The first element is coping, which refers to that space in time after experiencing adversity when you just take it moment by moment, hour by hour, day by day – before you are able to bounce forward. The Resilience Framework highlights both strategies and behaviours that can be adopted to help you cope. Putting on rose coloured glasses, being brave, remembering tomorrow is another day all seem superficial and phrases that you will have heard before, but in this element of the framework, they are key emotional and mindful mindsets that will support you in moving through this time.

Core self

The final element within the framework is core self. This element focuses on who you are. It recognises that you need to find ways to face problems and to find help when it is needed. It recognises this is a positive approach when trying to build a resilient spirt. At times this will involve you being hopeful despite the adversities that are being faced. It is having a sense of who you are and what you might need and acknowledging that becoming resilient will mean different things for different people.

Within the Resilience Framework (Figure 4.2), you will see four foundation stones of this approach are the noble truths. These truths are fundamental to most therapeutic approaches and are essential for the elements of the approach to have meaning. So, for example you need to be accepting of who you are, and this might mean that to develop your self-core you need to enlist the help of others. Later in the chapter you will be guided to think about the impact and value that applying this framework may have for you personally.

The Broaden and Build theory

Fredrickson (1998, 2001) developed a theory called the Broaden and Build theory. This theory suggests that positive emotions can account for differences in resilience. Fredrickson considers a psychological response to resilience and suggests that if an individual can focus on positive emotions, it can account for variances in personal levels of resilience. The theory suggests that positive emotions have the ability to not only reflect psychological resilience but also have the capacity to build it.

Figure 4.3 highlights how positive emotions build and broaden an individual's capacity to grow their resilience. It demonstrates how having a positive mindset is helpful in adversity.

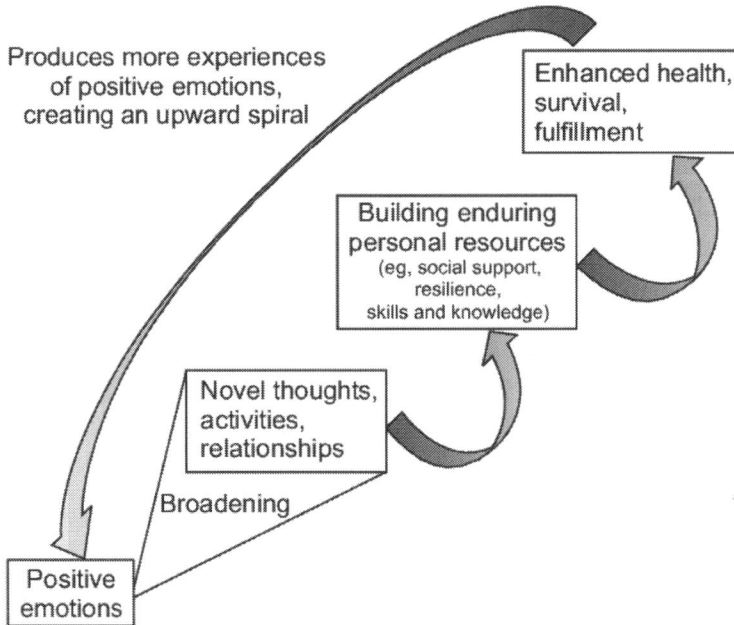

Figure 4.3 *The Broaden and Build theory, adapted from Fredrickson (1998, 2001)*

The Broaden and Build theory does not suggest you will not experience negative emotions since this is part of life. Instead, the theory suggests that if you are aware of, and build on positive emotions, you create a reserve that you can use when you experience negative emotions. For this approach to be affective, you will need to notice not only how positive emotions make you feel but also how they can affect all areas of your well-being and approach. Having this approach will have both an intrinsic effect and be extrinsically visible in your relationships with others. This, in turn, can build your support networks through having positive relationships with others as well as building an emotional reserve to use in times when you experience challenges in your personal and/or working life. The Broaden and Build theory has a cyclical nature which, as Figure 4.2 suggests, can lead to a more positive approach. As you read this you may be wondering how this might be achieved. It may be that its full effect cannot be seen until you have implemented strategies that can support you in thinking about how you build this reserve of positive emotions. This will be considered further in the concluding sections of the chapter.

CASE STUDY ⊖

Is this resilience?

Philippa had just secured a position as a manager of a nursery. At 25 she felt excited about this career promotion. In the first 6 months Philippa had worked hard to work alongside the team. She took the approach that managing in this way would help build trust and she hoped to build a sense of a shared vision for the setting. Staff meetings became places where ideas were shared, and where team members could share their thoughts on day-to-day practice.

The day the incident happened had been a usual morning – parents were dropping off their children and the nursey was bustling with the anticipation of all the Christmas events. Later in the morning a parent arrived and asked to speak to Philippa. She explained that she had come to share some sad news. Another parent who had left the nursery after dropping off had been killed in a road traffic accident. These children were at nursery, and she had come to collect them. At first Philippa felt a deep sense of shock about what she was hearing and how she could process the event. She could feel her body beginning to shake. There were so many thoughts moving through her head. But there was little time to process what was happening – she knew that she needed to be in the moment and support the parent who had come to collect the children. Quickly she collected the children from their homerooms within the nursery. They seemed excited to be being collected early and as Philippa helped them on with their coats, she felt a sense of deep sadness knowing that when they got home things would never be the same.

After they had left Philippa thought about how to share this news with the staff. She decided the only way was to tell the staff in smaller groups as the children still needed to be supervised. The staff were shocked and some of them had been working with the family for four years. One member of staff was really upset as she was one of the children's key person. She seemed angry – Philippa made her a tea, and they went into the garden. After a few moments the key person asked to be alone admitting that this was too much for her to handle having only lost her own father two months ago.

Philippa returned to her office; she too needed just a moment to collect her own thoughts. She remembered the death of her own grandparent as a child and how insecure she felt. How were they going to be able to support the children? How was she going to support everyone? Where could the team get support? She suddenly had the realisation that she needed to be with the team. Taking a few deep breaths Philippa joined the team. Everyone needed to pull together – the rest of the children were going to be collected soon. At the end of the day Philippa asked the team just to stay for a while, the kettle was put on and as a team they sat down together. Tears flowed, questions about how this could have happened were expressed and fears of how the team would or could support the children were expressed. As the door was closed to the nursery, Philippa thought about how in the morning she could have never imagined or wanted to experience a day like this.

Travelling to work the next day Philippa was nervous. How would she be able to hold it together? How was the team going to feel? Once at work the phone rang, the children who had lost their parents were on their way. The family felt that being at nursery would be good for them. The children arrived and went into their homerooms. After a while a member of staff who was working directly with one of the children said she was concerned as the child was taking the children into the home corner and telling the children that the parent had died. Philippa felt unsure about what to do; she tried to think about how could she bring something positive into this experience. Outside of work she had worked with children who had been bereaved, support had been given through Winston's Wish, a charity that supports children and their families who have experienced bereavement. Philippa wondered if phoning them would be helpful. She called and briefly explained what had happened. The support that she was given was clear and helpful; she was given advice on how to support the children, their family and the staff team. Philippa was asked about how she felt too, and it was good just for a moment to think about herself. Putting the phone down things felt better – there was something that could be done. Over the next few days, the team pulled together. This included talking with the children about what had happened and why the children who had lost their parent might feel sad. At the next staff meeting time was taken to talk about how this had felt. Staff were able to talk about the shock and how going through this had touched their own stories of bereavement. It was important to build on this experience for good. As a team they felt that there was a need to develop a bereavement policy within the nursery that would support the team in future practice.

Time to consider ☁

Before reflecting on the questions below, take a moment to think about some of the definitions and theories that have been considered. Can you see any theory in practice reflected within the scenario?

» How did Philippa show resilience in this scenario?

» In what ways did the team show trust in each other in this challenging situation?

» Thinking about both the Resilience Framework and the Broadening and Build theory, how did this scenario show aspects of both theories in practice?

» Earlier in the chapter we considered the notion of bouncing forward as a measure of a resilient spirit. How did the team show their desire to bounce forward?

Developing a personal resilience toolkit

In this concluding section, suggestions are made about how you might develop your own personal resilience tool kit. This is not a prescription but is a guide to suggestions that may be helpful. It might also be that reading this chapter has inspired some unique strategies that will support you.

Being aware of yourself

Throughout the chapter it has emerged that having an awareness of yourself, your body, your mind and your go-to reactions seem essential to being able to develop a resilient spirit. There are many ways in which you may try to do this. It could be that taking a walk somewhere that surrounds you with nature works and prompts feelings of joy. It could be that you enjoy yoga or meditation, a jog, or playing your favourite music. All are strategies that can prompt positive emotions, so the first step in building a resilient spirit is to answer the following questions.

- How can I give myself regular time to spend doing things that promote positive emotions within myself?

- If you know you don't do this, start by having one hour a week where you just do something that you enjoy – capture your thoughts at the end of this time.

Being aware of your go-to reactions in adversity

Part of being able to develop a resilient spirit or approach in adversity is becoming aware of yourself and knowing how you have reacted to adversity in the past.

- How might the HPA axis support you in accepting some of the reactions that you may have?

- Thinking about your reactions, how and what might help you when you are experiencing adversity both personally and within your work? If this involves gaining support from others or from your support networks, how can you develop this before challenges come your way?

Resilience health checks before, during and after challenges

Recognising that even with strategies and knowledge, sometimes we need to be resilient as things don't go to plan. It is therefore important when things are challenging, especially in a work situation, that you check in with your feelings and have an awareness of yourself.

- To support this, it is good practice when working in the sector to keep a journal where you reflect on practice but also record the positive strategies and go-to reactions as explored above. This will enable you to capture positive aspects of practice and solutions you can use when challenges arise. This way they are documented and available to use when we are stressed and less able to think straight.

- Alongside this, is it important to have a mentor in practice who you can share your thoughts with? (see Chapter 9).

- Finally, how can you bounce forward and what impact might this have on your professional identity and practice? For example, in the scenario explored the team decided to take their experience into practice development in the form of policy using the experience to enrich practice.

Chapter summary 📖

This chapter has explored what resilience might be. Having explored a variety of thinking it seems that there is no definitive definition of what resilience is. However, it appears that resilience can be developed within individuals where strategies, tools and an understanding of self are acknowledged. Exploring theories which promote resilience is a positive step in developing personal strategies that support practitioners to become more resilient as they work with children and their families.

Further reading 📚

Allies, S (2021) *Supporting Teacher Well-being: A Practical Guide for Primary Teachers and School Leaders.* Oxford: Routledge.

- This book is full of very practical ideas that promote a positive approach to developing well-being; this includes ideas that could have a big impact while in practice.

Neenan, M (2018) *Developing resilience: A Cognitive Behavioural Approach* Oxford: Routledge.

- This book digs deeper into the theories of resilience and throughout the book practical examples are given about how these could work in day-to-day life.

Zahariades, D (2020) *The Mental Toughness Handbook.* Art of Productivity.

- This is a book that is full of exercises and challenges that highlight strategies that could be helpful in developing resilience.

References 📚

Allies, S (2021) *Supporting Teacher Well-being: A Practical Guide for Primary Teachers and School Leaders* . Oxford: Routledge.

Barthélemy, E J, Thango, N S, Höhne, J, Lippa, L, Kolias, A, Task, W Y N F R and Germano, I M (2021) Resilience in the Face of the COVID-19 Pandemic: How to Bend and not Break. *World Neurosurgery,* 146: 280–4.

Blanden, J, Crawford, C, Drayton, E, Farquharson, C, Jarvie, M and Paull, G (2020) *Challenges for the Childcare Market: The Implications of COVID-19 for Childcare Providers in England.* London: The Institute for Fiscal Studies.

Edwards, E (2008) *Resilience: Reflections on the Burdens and Gifts of Facing Life's Adversities.* New York: Broadway Books.

Fletcher, D and Sarkar, M (2013) Psychological Resilience: A Review and Critique of Definitions, Concepts, and Theory. *European Psychologist,* 18(1): 12–23.

Fredrickson, B L (1998) What Good Are Positive Emotions? *Review of General Psychology*: Special Issue: New Directions in Research on Emotion. 1998; 2(3): 300–19.

Fredrickson, B L (2001) The Role of Positive Emotions in Positive Psychology: The Broaden-and-Build Theory of Positive Emotions. *American Psychologist*, 56(3): 218–26.

Grant, L and Kinman, G (2013) 'Bouncing Back?' Personal Representations of Resilience of Student and Experienced Social Workers. *Practice*, 25(5): 349–66.

Hart, A, Blincow, D and Thomas, H (2007) *Resilient Therapy: Working with Children and Families.* Hove: Routledge.

King, D D, Newman, A and Luthans, F (2016) Not If, but When We Need Resilience in the Workplace. *Journal of Organizational Behavior*, 37(5): 782–6.

Mu, M (2021) Sociologising Resilience through Bourdieu's Field Analysis: Misconceptualisation, Conceptualisation, and Reconceptualization. *British Journal of Sociology of Education*, 42(1):15–31.

Neenan, M (2018) *Developing Resilience: A Cognitive Behavioural Approach.* Oxford: Routledge.

Rajan-Rankin, S (2014) Self-identity, Embodiment and the Development of Emotional Resilience. *The British Journal of Social Work*, 44(8): 2426–42.

Rose, S and Palattiyil, G (2020) Surviving or Thriving? Enhancing the Emotional Resilience of Social Workers in their Organisational Settings. *Journal of Social Work*, 20(1): 23–42.

Tugade, M M and Fredrickson, B L (2004) Resilient Individuals Use Positive Emotions to Bounce Back from Negative Emotional Experiences. *Journal of Personality and Social Psychology*, 86(2): 320–33.

Walsh, F (2016) *Strengthening Family Resilience* (3rd ed). New York: Guildford Press.

5 Empathy, compassion and emotion

ANGELA HODGKINS

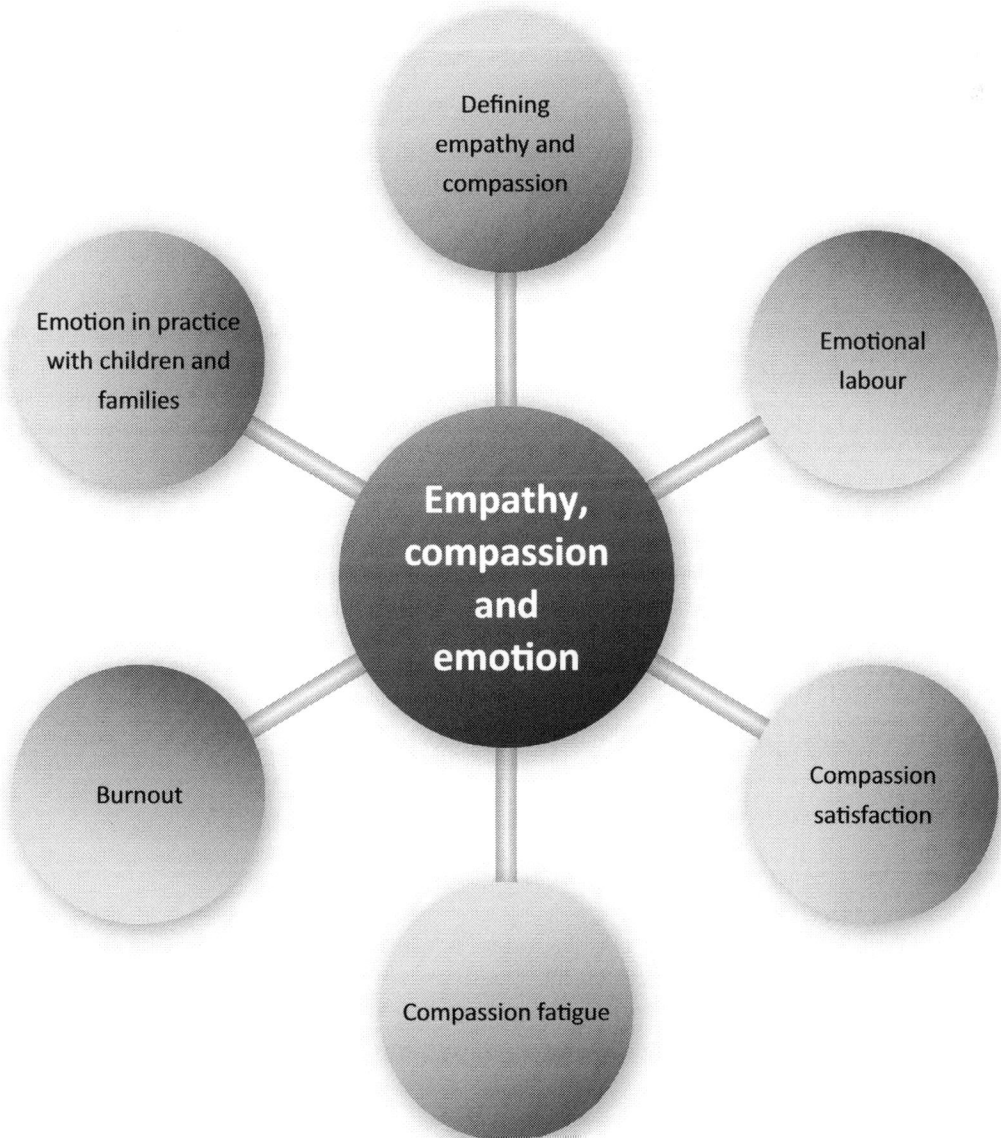

Chapter objectives ◎

This chapter enables you to reflect on your experience of empathy, compassion and emotion within practice with children and families. The chapter:

- defines empathy and compassion within practice;
- investigates 'empathic distress', 'compassion fatigue' and burnout;
- explores 'compassion satisfaction' and personal fulfilment;
- examines 'emotional labour' and the impact on the practitioner.

Critical questions ⑦

» How would you define empathy and compassion?

» What do you consider to be the emotional impact of your role?

» What led to you choosing a career working with children and families?

Introduction

Most people would agree that anyone working with children and families should be empathic and compassionate, but it is not always clear what this means in practice, how you can develop and demonstrate these skills, and what the impact of this highly emotional work might be on the practitioner. The aim of this chapter is to define terms and to examine types of empathy and different responses to it, one being compassion and the other 'empathic distress'. We will examine what this is, how it can lead to burnout and how to avoid this. It is also important to examine the positive effects of empathy which can result in job satisfaction, and the passion to make a difference that endures within the profession. The 'emotional labour' involved in the profession is not always acknowledged, so the chapter will also examine the implications of this for practice.

Defining empathy

One of the first writers to define empathy as a skill was Carl Rogers, who defined it as being able to understand how another person may be feeling, to see the world through the service user's eyes, '*to sense the client's private world as if it were your own*' (Rogers, 1957, p 96). Rogers' writing was about empathy in relation to counselling therapy, but he asserted that the skill was equally important for anyone working with people.

The literature regarding stages of empathy can be confusing, as there is no one explanation that is agreed by all writers. Anyone working with young children will know that empathy develops as we grow and learn. Primitive empathy is a very basic, non-conscious form of empathy. Have you ever noticed that when another person yawns, you yawn too? Or that when a baby cries in the nursery, others cry too? This is primitive empathy; it is an automatic emotional response that requires no conscious thought. Later, the capacity to understand other people's emotional states, often referred to as 'theory of mind' develops. There is much academic debate about when children develop 'theory of mind'. Traditional theorists believe that it starts from four years of age (Westby and Robinson, 2014), but some contemporary theorists believe that it starts much earlier, from around 15 months (Gopnik, 2010). Theory of mind includes being able to understand both your own and another person's emotions and being able to imagine how things feel for others. Another, more complex, form is '*advanced empathy*' (Egan, 2013). This composite skill involves tuning in to the other person, picking up on unspoken signs such as body language and being aware of feelings that the other person may not be conscious of. There is evidence to suggest that this advanced form of empathy is what practitioners may be demonstrating in their work with young children (Hodgkins, 2019).

Affective versus cognitive empathy

The two central views on types of empathy are the affective tradition and the cognitive tradition. A third view, the multidimensional approach, recognises that both affective and cognitive empathy are required in caring professions.

Table 5.1 *Types of empathy*

Affective empathy	Cognitive empathy	Multidimensional empathy
Experiencing the emotion of another person oneself	Rational understanding of another person's feelings	An emotional response, followed by a response resulting from cognition
'Picking up' on the emotions of others, so that you start to experience the same emotion	Closely related to 'theory of mind' – the ability to consider what a situation is like from someone else's point of view	*Caring* professionals need to demonstrate both types of empathy in their role
Affective empathy is more important because it helps us to build social relationships (Maibom, 2017)	Cognitive empathy is more important because it involves intellectual reasoning (Decety and Yoder, 2016)	The emotional effect is a key concept, but it should be followed by a response resulting from some form of cognitive activity (Eisenberg et al, 1991)
Example – a friend's cat has been killed in a road accident. She is devastated and I feel devastated too.	Example – a friend has failed his driving test for the third time. He is very upset, so I try to think about how he must be feeling and what he might need from me.	Example – a friend is in hospital waiting for surgery and is feeling anxious. I pick up on her anxiety and feel anxious for her, so I think about what would help me in that situation and I send her funny messages to take her mind off the wait.

> ***Time to consider***
>
> »   List five times that you have expressed empathy within your practice. Now reflect on the types of empathy above (Table 5.1) and try to ascertain which type(s) of empathy you have experienced.

There has been very little research conducted into types of empathy used by children and families' practitioners, but there have been publications based on types of empathy in nursing and in social work. An article by Morse et al (1991) examining empathy in nurses concluded that emotional empathy followed by a professional response is the essence of a nurse–patient relationship. This constitutes a multidimensional view of empathy which is mirrored in research by Gerdes and Segal (2009) who examined empathy skills for social workers. They suggested that what is required is a three-stage process, an affective response to another's emotion, cognitive processing and then cognitive decision-making.

Developing empathy skills

Empathy skills develop throughout childhood, from the earliest examples of infants wanting to comfort others in distress at around 12 months to the regulation of children's own emotions which develops into adolescence. There is a view that empathy is a personal quality, that one is either an empathic person or not (Ratka, 2018), but there is ample literature suggesting that empathy is a skill that can be taught, learned and developed. Morse et al (1991, p 82) assert that affective empathy, '*reading people's needs and knowing implicitly what to do*' when someone is in distress, is gained from experience and modelling by more experienced professionals.

Empathic understanding can be developed in adulthood by exposure to other people. Talking to others, especially people with very different lives and experiences and watching TV programmes about people whose experiences are different from your own is a good way of increasing your ability to put yourself in other people's position. Listening to others is equally, or more, important, so practising 'active listening' skills will also help you to understand the experiences of others. Learning about body language and facial expressions can be very useful in increasing your ability to be able to '*read*' non-verbal clues (Svinth, 2018). Advanced empathy skills rely heavily on this skill to empathise with others' unspoken emotions (Egan, 2010). Baron-Cohen et al (2001) devised the '*reading the mind in the eyes*' test to measure theory of mind. Baron-Cohen's adapted version (2009) which looks at the faces of children was designed to help identify Autism in children, but it is useful in assessing your own empathic skills.

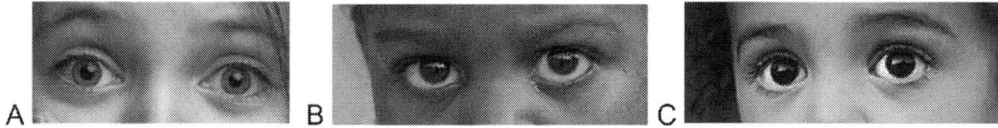
Compassion

Although sometimes used synonymously, empathy and compassion are different concepts. Empathy refers to the sharing of emotions with others, whereas compassion is an active concept, something that is demonstrated, often as a result of empathy. Most children and families' practitioners consider themselves as compassionate and there is much evidence to support this view. Taggart (2016, p 176) defines compassion as '*alleviating suffering, vulnerability and inequality … whilst calling on personal emotions for their motivation*'. The children in our settings are sometimes suffering, often vulnerable, and sometimes treated unequally, so compassionate practice is what they need from those caring for them. Dachyshyn (2015, 36–7) suggests that when we are non-judgemental and respond to children compassionately, '*from the heart*', then we create a close and mindful relationship that encourages them to grow into compassionate adults.

Emotional labour

The term 'emotional labour' refers to the suppression or demonstration of your emotions. In Hochschild's (1983, p 7) book, she defined it as '*the management of feeling to create a publicly observable facial and bodily display*'. Hochschild's research began with airline cabin crew, who are expected to cover up any feelings of frustration, irritability or tiredness in order to provide good customer service, despite the research uncovering some very difficult situations that they have to endure, including smiling through racist comments from passengers. Hochschild (2012, p 50) believes that this 'commercialisation of feelings', the suppression of emotion and the requirement to express appropriate emotions for the job role can be very emotionally draining. Hochschild lists the early childhood profession as one where emotional labour is expected and there is much research suggesting that this is a very significant factor. There is a gender influence, too, with many of the workforces that rely on emotional labour being predominantly female. Page and Elfer (2013, p 553) researched attachment in a nursery environment and identified evidence of 'the emotional demands on staff of sustaining' practice with children and their families, from interactions with children, parents and other professionals.

Empathic distress and compassion fatigue

As discussed earlier, empathy can have both positive and negative consequences. Hoffman (2000) believes that affective empathy, feeling the distress of others, causes us to feel distressed ourselves; this is known as 'empathic distress'. Eisenberg (2005) calls it 'empathic over-arousal' which, if not managed effectively, can result in stress and burnout. There is lots of evidence from research in caring professions that empathy can cause distress (Bry et al, 2016; Motthagi et al, 2019; Lynch et al, 2019), although this may be only in particularly susceptible individuals (Tone and Tully, 2014).

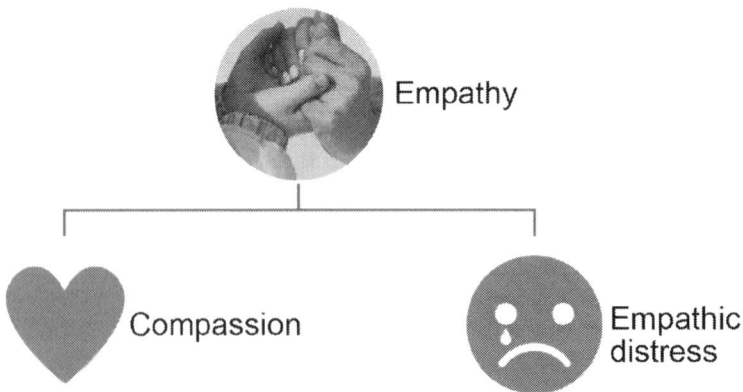

Figure 5.2 *Consequences of empathy*

'Compassion fatigue' is another term for the same phenomenon, as is 'secondary trauma', a term describing the trauma we feel personally if we are around someone going through a traumatic event. Compassion fatigue appears to be an accepted occupational hazard for those working in caring professions. There is a view that practitioners have a vocation, a selfless desire to help and put others' feelings before their own. In Elfer et al's (2018) article on 'Love, satisfaction and exhaustion in the nursery', the writers outline examples of the sorts of things that can lead to compassion fatigue: witnessing children's difficult separation from their parent, coping with children's overwhelming emotions, and working with children experiencing mental health difficulties, bereavement and family breakdown. Datler et al (2010, p 82) describe '*how hard and disturbing it is, to be confronted so intimately with the ... often catastrophic emotions of very young children*'. A recent report by Nelinger et al (2021) uncovered some alarming statistics from nursery workers in the UK:

*   69 per cent of them had worked with babies or children suffering from trauma or abuse;

*   71 per cent had worked with babies or children affected by domestic violence;

*   91 per cent said they had dealt with challenging situations involving mental health, social or emotional difficulties;

*   71 per cent said they had been stressed or upset;

*   74 per cent said they felt unsure of the best way to deal with difficult situations.

With so many practitioners struggling to manage difficult situations, and the age old problems with feeling undervalued by society (Jovanovic, 2013), compassion fatigue seems a high risk.

Burnout

Burnout is defined by the World Health Organization (2019) as '*a syndrome conceptualized as resulting from chronic workplace stress that has not been successfully managed*'. Therefore, burnout can be understood as the extreme form of empathic distress or unresolved compassion fatigue. Burnout is characterised by exhaustion, negative feelings, reduced work performance and detachment from the role. When practitioners can no longer cope with the amount of stress they are confronted with, they can withdraw and become remote and cold. Burnout can also lead to physical symptoms such as insomnia, heart problems, susceptibility to infection, depression, and a reliance on alcohol or other negative coping mechanisms. It is vital to develop positive self-care strategies in order to protect oneself from burnout.

To prevent burnout, it is important to reflect on your work and your mental state. Reflective practice can help to identify areas of work that are problematic. Roberts et al (2019) suggest that practitioners who practice reflective writing in particular are less likely to experience burnout. Reflection can help to identify unreasonable demands and unmanageable workloads. If this is the case, then it is important to talk this through with someone. Talking to managers or personnel staff will enable employers to support workers through difficulties and so reduce any significant effects on mental or physical health. Elfer (2012) advocates regular discussions on the emotional experiences within the early childhood workplace, focusing on helping the staff team to reflect on and manage these emotional interactions (see Chapters 2 and 3).

Compassion satisfaction

It is important to acknowledge that while there is considerable compassion fatigue within the children and families sector, there is also significant satisfaction in the role. Stamm (1996) wrote about the importance of measuring compassion satisfaction as well as compassion fatigue. Stamm agrees with the notion that empathy results in taking action and showing compassion and there is evidence to suggest that when we take action, this can help us to feel less distressed, so we feel better if we can help. A good example of this is when we see terrible upsetting stories on the news; if we donate some money to the cause, we feel better. Hansen et al (2018) suggest that, although in the short term, empathy can result in compassion fatigue, in the long term it can result in compassion satisfaction. Thus, if one feels exhausted or fatigued at the end of the day, looking back on the overall experience of working with children brings satisfaction. Elfer et al's (2018) research on work discussion suggests that this would not only reduce compassion fatigue but also increase satisfaction. Andreychik (2019) asserts that while strong and repeated connection with others' negative emotions can place individuals at greater risk for burnout, connecting with others' positive emotions may help protect against burnout and increase job satisfaction.

Critical questions ⑦

» What can you do within your work environment to encourage the '*connection with others' positive emotions*' that Andreychik (2019) recommends?

» What opportunities are there within the workplace to share a laugh, to celebrate good times and achievements? How might this be improved in your workplace?

Spotlight on new debates

Empathy bias

New research on empathy bias exposes questions about whether empathy is always constructive and positive. There have been suggestions in past research that empathy may involve bias, that we are more likely to feel empathy towards people who are similar to us in some way, for example, racially, socially and culturally (Prinz, 2011; Bloom, 2016). In Bloom's (2016) book, '*Against empathy*', he calls for '*rational compassion*' rather than emotional empathy which he believes is a poor guide for making decisions. There has been a long debate about how much emotion affects decision-making.

Fowler et al (2021) conducted research into empathy bias with 300 members of the public who completed an anonymous online questionnaire. Participants were shown short descriptions of people and situations. They then had to make moral judgements about the scenarios and clarify the amount of empathy they felt. The study found that people are more likely to feel empathy for others who are close to us socially. However, the study also found that participants thought that it was important to show empathy equally to all. It seems, therefore, that although we agree that empathy is important, there is some unconscious bias in our responses. In contrast, Read (2021) suggests that this is not the case, since empathy can help us to understand people with opposing moral, social and political views to our own. This, she says, is why it is so important in helping us to handle disagreements and see the other person's point of view. It is possible that Read (2021) is considering cognitive empathy here.

CASE STUDY ⊖

Empathy in the time of a worldwide pandemic

A current research project (Hodgkins, 2021) has uncovered significant effects of the recent Covid-19 pandemic on the emotional well-being of practitioners in the UK. The project's aim was to examine perceptions of empathy within the role of early years practitioners from a range of early years settings. Participants were asked to complete a reflective diary, focusing on empathic interactions within their role, followed by an interview to further discuss some of their entries. Interim findings have exposed examples of emotional and sometimes distressing interactions with children, resulting in many practitioners struggling to cope. Excerpts from the diaries are identified here in *italics*. Participants expressed concern over the regression they have seen in children now that they are returning to nursery after the national lockdowns. This is particularly noticeable in relation to self-care, with children having to re-learn skills such as putting on their own coats and shoes when returning to nursery. Practitioners describe children struggling with the transition to the setting and having to build attachments, '*as if they have had to start over again*'. One participant said, '*Children seem overwhelmed by the change and unused to being in a noisy group of people*' and another expressed how difficult it was for her to see very young children suffering with anxiety. Practitioners have also had to deal with increased anxiety from parents and carers, one participant describing the added pressure of having worried parents and carers fretting and constantly phoning to check on their child. This added tension has exacerbated the stress levels in a profession already endeavouring to manage the emotional labour involved in their work. Many early years practitioners have been working harder than ever during the pandemic, caring for some of the most disadvantaged children in very difficult conditions. The emotional cost is expressed in comments such as these: '*I do really struggle at work a lot of the time; it's been so draining emotionally, I'm constantly thinking about work, especially safeguarding issues*'; '*I feel a sense of responsibility and that causes me to overthink and be anxious and sometimes not be able to sleep*'; '*it's getting more emotionally taxing; I do think about a lot of the children when I'm not at work*'.

Despite this emotional overload and the difficulties in managing unsettled children and anxious families, early years practitioners are committed to doing their very best for the children in their care and they are supporting each other as best they can. One participant in the research said, '*the staff all support each other; we cry together over something most days*'.

Time to consider ☁

Now that you have read the case study above, reflect on the following.

» Do these examples of practice seem familiar? Have you experienced similar things?

» How well can you balance compassion fatigue with compassion satisfaction?

> » One of the participants said, '*we cry together over something most days*'; is this ok? What are the consequences of this level of emotional labour?
>
> » How would you know if you were in danger of experiencing burnout? What would you do?
>
> » What can you learn from this chapter for yourself and your practice?

Chapter summary

In this chapter, we have examined definitions of empathy and how this differs from compassion. We have considered affective and cognitive empathy and ways that these types of empathy might impact on us as practitioners. We have explored both compassion fatigue and compassion satisfaction and looked at ways of preventing burnout in our practice. We have also investigated some current research into empathy and a case study that aims to analyse empathy within early years practice.

In conclusion, empathy is an essential element of working with young children, it makes us compassionate and it helps us to build the close relationships which are so important in our profession.

Answers to the Baron-Cohen facial expression test: A – panicked; B – serious; C – thoughtful.

Further reading

Bloom, P (2016) *Against Empathy: The Case for Rational Compassion*. London: Penguin.

• This book is not, as it suggests, a book suggesting that we do not use empathy. It calls for 'rational compassion' as opposed to biased emotional empathy.

Howe, D (2013) *Empathy: What It Is and Why It Matters*. Basingstoke: Palgrave Macmillan.

• A book all about aspects of empathy for those who want to find out much more.

Solvason, C, Hodgkins, A and Watson, N (2020) Preparing Students for the 'Emotion Work' of Early Years Practice. *NZ International Research in Early Childhood Education Journal*, 23(1): 14–23.

• This article outlines the emotional aspect of working with young children and suggests ways of preparing practitioners for this.

References

Andreychik, M (2019) Feeling Your Joy Helps Me to Bear Feeling Your Pain: Examining Associations between Empathy for Others' Positive versus Negative Emotions and Burnout. *Personality and Individual Differences*, 137: 147–56.

Baron-Cohen, S (2009) The Empathising-Systemising Theory of Autism: Implications for Education. *Tizard Learning Disability Review*, 14(3): 4–13.

Baron-Cohen, S, Wheelwright, S, Hill, J, Raste, Y and Plumb, I (2001) The 'Reading the Mind in the Eyes' Test Revised Version: A Study with Normal Adults, and Adults with Asperger Syndrome or High-functioning Autism. *Journal of Child Psychology and Psychiatry*, 42(2): 241–51.

Bloom, P (2016) *Against Empathy: The Case for Rational Compassion*. London: Penguin.

Bry, K, Bry, M, Hentz, E, Karlsson, H L, Kyllönen, H, Lundkvist, M and Wigert, H (2016) Communication Skills Training Enhances Nurses' Ability to Respond with Empathy to Parents' Emotions in a Neonatal Intensive Care Unit. *Acta Paediatrica*, 105(4): 397–406.

Dachyshyn, D M (2015) Being Mindful, Heartful, and Ecological in Early Years Care and Education. *Contemporary Issues in Early Childhood*, 16(1): 32–41.

Datler, W, Datler, M and Funder, A (2010) Struggling against a Feeling of Becoming Lost: A Young Boy's Painful Transition to Day Care. *Infant Observation*, 13(1): 65–87.

Decety, J and Yoder, K J (2016) Empathy and Motivation for Justice: Cognitive Empathy and Concern, but not Emotional Empathy, Predict Sensitivity to Injustice for Others. *Social Neuroscience*, 11(1): 1–14.

Egan, G (2010) *The Skilled Helper: A Problem-Management and Opportunity-Development Approach to Helping* (9th ed). Pacific Grove, CA: Brooks Cole.

Egan, G (2013) *The Skilled Helper: A Problem-Management and Opportunity-Development Approach to Helping* (10th ed). Pacific Grove, CA: Brooks Cole.

Eisenberg, N, Shea, C L, Carlo, G and Knight, G P (1991) Empathy-related Responding and Cognition: A 'Chicken and the Egg' Dilemma. In Kurtines, W M and Gewirtz, J L (eds) *Handbook of Moral Behavior and Development, Vol. 2: Research* (pp 63–88). Hillsdale: Lawrence Erlbaum Associates.

Elfer, P (2012) Emotion in Nursery Work: Work Discussion as a Model of Critical Professional Reflection. *Early Years*, 32(2): 129–41.

Elfer, P, Greenfield, S, Robson, S, Wilson, D and Zachariou, A (2018) Love, Satisfaction and Exhaustion in the Nursery: Methodological Issues in Evaluating the Impact of Work Discussion Groups in the Nursery. *Early Child Development and Care*, 188(7): 892–904.

Fowler, Z, Fiore-Law, K and Gaesser, B (2021) Against Empathy Bias: The Moral Value of Equitable Empathy. *Association for Psychological Science*, 32(5): 766–79.

Gerdes, K and Segal, E (2009) A Social Work Model of Empathy. *Advances in Social Work*, 10(2): 114–27.

Gopnik, A (2010) How Babies Think. *Scientific American*, 303: 76–81.

Hansen, E, Hakansson Eklund, J, Hallen, A, Stockman Bjurhager, C, Norrstrom, E, Viman, A and Stocks, E (2018) Does Feeling Empathy Lead to Compassion Fatigue or Compassion Satisfaction? The Role of Time Perspective. *The Journal of Psychology,* 152(8): 630–45.

Hochschild, A (1983) *The Managed Heart: Commercialization of Human Feeling*. Berkeley, CA: University of California Press.

Hochschild, A (2012) *The Managed Heart: Commercialization of Human Feeling*. California: University of California Press.

Hodgkins, A (2019) Advanced Empathy in the Early Years – A Risky Strength? *NZ International Research in Early Childhood Education Journal*, 22(1): 46–58.

Hodgkins, A (2021) Early Years Practitioners Need Emotional Support Too. *Nursery Management Today*, 21(2): 33.

Hoffman, M L (2000) *Empathy and Moral Development: Implications for Caring and Justice.* Cambridge: Cambridge University Press.

Jovanovic, J (2013), Retaining Early Childcare Educators. *Gender, Work and Organisation*, 20(5): 528–44.

Lynch, A, Newlands, F and Forrester, D (2019) What Does Empathy Sound Like in Social Work Communication? A Mixed-methods Study of Empathy in Child Protection Social Work Practice. *Child & Family Social Work*, 24(1): 139–47.

Maibom, H (2017) *The Routledge Handbook of Philosophy of Empathy.* New York: Routledge.

Morse, J M, Bottorff, J, Anderson, G, O'Brien, B and Solberg, S (2006) Beyond Empathy: Expanding Expressions of Caring. *Journal of Advanced Nursing*, 53(1): 75–87.

Motthagi, S, Poursheikhali, H and Shameli, L (2019) Empathy, Compassion Fatigue, Guilt and Secondary Traumatic Stress in Nurses. *Nursing Ethics*, 1(1): 96–7.

Nelinger, A, Album, J, Haynes, A and Rosan, C (2021) Their Challenges Are Our Challenges. *Anna Freud National Centre for Children and Families*. [online] Available at: www.annafreud.org (accessed 27 July 2021).

Page, J and Elfer, P (2013) The Emotional Complexity of Attachment Interactions in Nursery. *European Early Childhood Education Research Journal*, 21(4): 553–67.

Prinz, J (2011) Against Empathy. *Southern Journal of Philosophy*, 49(1): 214–33.

Ratka, A (2018) Empathy and the Development of Affective Skills. *American Journal of Pharmaceutical Education*, 82(10): 7192.

Read, H (2021) Empathy and Common Ground. *Ethical Theory and Moral Practice*, 24: 459–73.

Roberts, A, LoCasale-Crouch, J, Hamre, B and Jamil, F (2020) Preschool Teachers' Self-efficacy, Burnout, and Stress in Online Professional Development: A Mixed Methods Approach to Understand Change. *Journal of Early Childhood Teacher Education*, 41(3): 262–83.

Rogers, C R (1957) The necessary and sufficient conditions of therapeutic personality change. *Journal of Consulting and Clinical Psychology*, 21(2): 95–103.

Stamm, B H (2002) Measuring Compassion Satisfaction as well as Fatigue: Developmental History of the Compassion Satisfaction and Fatigue Test. In Figley C R (ed) *Treating Compassion Fatigue* (107–19). New York: Brunner-Routledge.

Svinth, L (2018) Being Touched – The Transformative Potential of Nurturing Touch Practices in Relation to Toddlers' Learning and Emotional Well-being. *Early Child Development and Care*, 188(7): 924–36.

Taggart, G (2016) Compassionate Pedagogy: The Ethics of Care in Early Childhood Professionalism. *European Early Childhood Education Research Journal*, 24(2): 173–85.

Tone, E and Tully, E (2014) Empathy as a 'Risky Strength': A Multilevel Examination of Empathy and Risk for Internalizing Disorders. *Development and Psychopathology*, 26(4pt2): 1547–65.

Westby, C and Robinson, L (2014) A Developmental Perspective for Promoting Theory of Mind. *Topics in Language Disorders*, 34(4): 362–83.

World Health Organization (2019) Burn-out an 'Occupational Phenomenon': International Classification of Diseases. [online] Available at www.who.int/news/item/28-05-2019-burn-out-an-occupational-phenomenon-international-classification-of-diseases (accessed 27 July 2021).

Part 3 Succeeding amid work-based learning issues

6 Finding your place in safeguarding practice

MICHELLE MALOMO AND EMMA LAURENCE

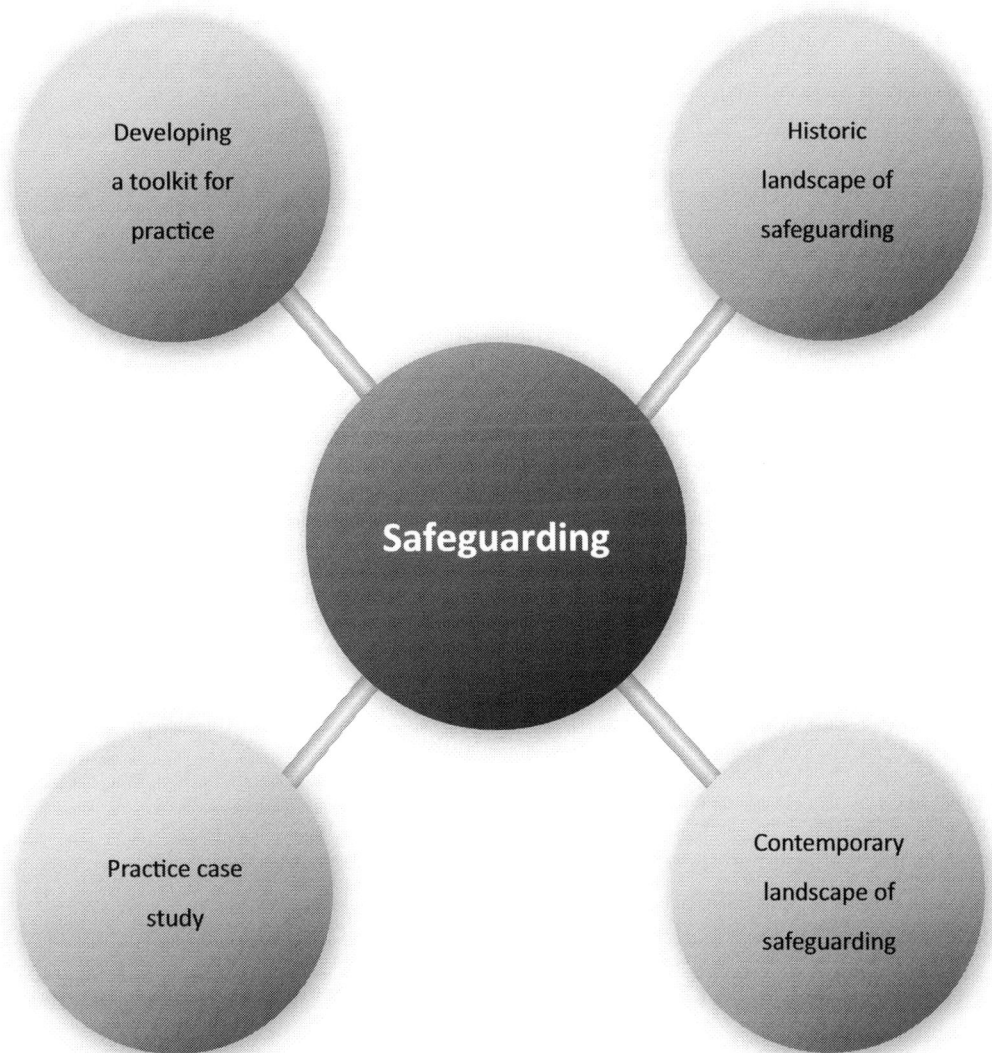

Developing a toolkit for practice

Historic landscape of safeguarding

Safeguarding

Practice case study

Contemporary landscape of safeguarding

Chapter objectives ◎

Safeguarding and keeping safe is a central aspect of child and family support work. This chapter therefore encourages the reader to engage critically in the formation of cultures of vigilance within the sector. It supports the reader to reflect on subjects such as: what constitutes a safe place to work; emotional safety; being 'covid-secure' and indeed what security might mean in a time of insecurity. It aims to equip you to understand how to safeguard the relationship with the host setting and to take advantage of opportunities to learn through reflective practice so that they can make a critical contribution to inter-agency practice. This chapter:

- gives an overview of the landscape of safeguarding in the UK;
- supports those working in the children and families' sector in locating themselves within this sector;
- develops an understanding of new debates in the safeguarding arena;
- provides tools to support the personal development of attributes such as courage and finding your own voice.

Introduction

At the start of this chapter, it is important to gain an understanding as to how safeguarding practice has developed over time. The chapter starts by exploring the historic and contemporary landscapes of safeguarding, as this will help you to explore and gain a deeper understanding of practice. Having this understanding supports informed practice. However, when we are working to safeguard children, we may become so focused on procedures and processes that the experiences and theories that shape our practice are forgotten. The chapter is mindful of and addresses this point.

The historic landscape of safeguarding

As soon as you set foot in a setting, there is the potential to be overwhelmed by the dos, don'ts and absolutely musts of policy in this arena. As a well-intended trainee practitioner this can feel like an initiation process meant to intimidate. Actually, however, it is indicative of the statutory position that the 'child's welfare is paramount'. Therefore, the first and foremost responsibility for your in-setting mentor is to ensure that you have a thorough understanding of your safeguarding responsibilities in setting.

It is easy at this stage in your career to see yourself as adjacent to professionals in setting, working parallel to, rather than within, an integrated team. Often student practitioners wait in the wings for instruction. Understandably tentative and all the while observing good practice, the student practitioner often participates where they feel confident to do so. However, when it comes to safeguarding and protecting children, there is no room for hesitation or assuming those more qualified are acting on a concern. '*Everyone who works with children has a responsibility for keeping them safe*' (HM Government 2018, p 11).

Safeguarding is a relatively new area of legislation within the UK with the prevention of Cruelty to Animals Act (1876) preceding the development of the Prevention of Cruelty to Children Act (1889). Up until the late nineteenth century, the government had little inclination to interfere in the home life of families. Powell and Uppal (2012) highlight that the introduction of societies for the prevention of cruelty to children (such as the NSPCC) in the late nineteenth century was underpinned by new child protection legislation. This arrived first in the United States before arriving in the UK. In the United States, this seemed to follow the case of Mary Ellen Wilson, who in 1872 was ultimately removed from an abusive situation thanks to the actions of a 'concerned citizen' who recognised the signs of ill-treatment and acted accordingly (Myers, 2004). Due to the public interest in the media coverage of this case, awareness of child protection issues grew. Within safeguarding contexts, the concerned individual pursuing the interests of the child remains pivotal today.

Legislative responses to the lessons learned from the individual cases reveal a pattern that is common across the history of safeguarding and child protection practices. However, the cases which have impacted legislation and practice most often arise from public inquiry into the death or serious harm of children. This means that the greatest focus is upon 'what went wrong' and examples of good practice rarely inspire legislation in this arena. Perhaps the most pivotal case to impact upon safeguarding legislation is that of Victoria Climbié (1991–2000). Following her death at the hands of her great-aunt and her great-aunt's boyfriend in 2000, an inquiry was set up, chaired by Lord Laming. In total, the report yielded 108 recommendations that impacted professional practice and legislation within the children and families' sector enormously. Particularly pertinent was the development of Every Child Matters (DfES, 2003) which focused on improving services for children and families through greater accountability and service reform. Every Child Matters (2003) placed the whole child at the centre of practice with the idea that services, such as health, education and care, would become more integrated.

In addition to understanding the legislative requirements of professionals who work with children and families, Lord Laming's report also touches on a more specific element of practice which this chapter seeks to promote. At the beginning of the report, he identifies the skills and qualities required of those working with children, stating:

> I recognize that those who take on the work of protecting children at risk of deliberate harm face a tough and challenging task. Staff doing this work need a combination of professional skills and personal qualities, not least of which are **persistence** and **courage**.
>
> (Laming, 2003, p 3)

While the role you hold in protecting children can feel like a daunting one, it is important to remember that you are not alone in this. As a professional, you, along with collaborating staff members of your setting, constitute a wider community around the child, serving as a safety net in protecting them. It is everyone's duty to play a role in this. It is easier to feel courageous when you lean into this team, making it important to ensure there are strong lines of communication between you and the professionals around you. Upon arrival it is essential to identify and get to know who the Designated Safeguarding Lead (DSL) in setting is as they are your point of contact on issues of child welfare and child protection. According to the Statutory Guidance for Schools (Department for Education, 2021, p 8), the task of the DSL is to *'provide support to staff to carry out their safeguarding duties'*. Crucial also is the understanding that the importance of confidentiality cannot come at the cost of a timely response. Sharing only with 'those that need to know' is not supposed to pose a barrier to appropriate care in the name of confidentiality; rather this principle includes those that help you in acting on concerns appropriately. For example, within the statutory guidance (DfE, 2021, p 18) it states that while the role of the DSL is to always be available to support staff, in exceptional circumstances when this is not possible *'staff should consider speaking to a member of the senior leadership team and/or take advice from local children's social care'*, reporting back to the DSL as soon as is practicably possible.

Time to consider ☁

» Reflect on how legislation has been created over time. Do you notice any patterns in the events that have served as catalysts in creating policy change?

» How do you think these trends could impact upon the policy that follows?

The contemporary landscape of safeguarding

Earlier the chapter highlighted that the Laming enquiry (2003) recognised being part of the safeguarding landscape requires persistence and courage. To be able to develop this approach in line with current thinking, it is important to have an understanding of the contemporary landscape of safeguarding. This will support you in gaining confidence in developing your practice in this area.

In recent years, the landscape of safeguarding in England has been influenced by the need to hold someone accountable for mistakes that have been made when trying to safeguard children. There have been numerous Serious Case Reviews (SCR) associated with named children. This has heightened media attention in these cases, where the purpose seems to have been to apportion blame for what went wrong and where accountability has been central to government policy. Frost (2021, p 32) suggests that this is both *'negative and damaging'* and fails to recognise much of the success of multi-agency working. The government has wanted to be seen to be accountable and has commissioned two significant reviews: Munro (DfE, 2011) and Wood (2016). Alongside these reviews there have been several iterations of the *Working Together to Safeguard Children* guidance (HM Government, 2018). To support your practice development, it is important to understand these documents and how they shape your responsibilities and practice within the contemporary safeguarding landscape.

The Munro review of child protection: a child-centred system (2011)

This was commissioned by the then Secretary of State for Education and at its heart had the question *'What helps professionals make the best judgments they can to protect a vulnerable child?'*. The findings of this review recommended the need to move away from the over-bureaucratised systems that focused on administrative compliance *'to one that values and develops professional expertise and is focused on the safety and welfare of children and young people*' (Munro, 2011, p 9). Gallagher and Sutton-Tsang (2017) suggest an important outcome of the Munro report is that it is essential that practitioners develop practice that reflects Munro's call for a learning culture within safeguarding practice. This involves practice that seeks to 'do the right thing' when safeguarding children rather than just 'doing things right' bureaucratically. The recommendations within this report also highlight the importance of early help and specialised training for social workers and recommended a review of how Local Safeguarding Children's Boards (LSCB) were operating.

Wood report: review of the role and functions of local safeguarding children boards (2016)

This review made some significant changes and builds on the findings of Munro. In summary it suggested that LSCBs should be abolished and replaced with three lead safeguarding partners working together to safeguard children (local authorities, chief officer of the police and clinical commissioning groups). These safeguarding partners will identify and arrange the review of SCRs and think about the issues that have been raised within these for their area. The review also suggested that a National Child Safeguarding Practice Review Panel should be established to publish the outcomes of reviews of child safeguarding practice.

Working together to safeguard children (2018)

The final guidance that has shaped the practice within the contemporary landscape is the Working together to safeguard children (2018) guidance. This outlines the government's guidance for all in safeguarding children. It states:

> *Everyone who works with children has a responsibility for keeping them safe. No single practitioner can have a full picture of a child's needs and circumstances and, if children and families are to receive the right help at the right time, everyone who comes into contact with them has a role to play in identifying concerns, sharing information and taking prompt action.*
>
> (HMG, 2018, p 11)

Gallagher and Sutton-Tsang (2017) explore this responsibility and suggest the danger of accepting that this is everyone's responsibility may cause you to think someone else is responding to concerns, as after all it is everyone's responsibility. Or you respond at the opposite end of the spectrum where every child you come into contact with is your responsibility and you must be responsible for their well-being. Gallagher and Sutton-Tsang (2017, p 161) suggest that it is important to develop practice that supports us to be '*active, effectively contributing to young children's lives in a way that helps children's well-being and welfare ... in short it prepares us to be vigilant and not a vigilante*'. This insight is helpful when as a practitioner you are developing your thinking and practice in this area.

To support you in this it is important that you have a good, secure knowledge and understanding of current guidance. Throughout Working together to safeguard children (2018), practice is driven by an understanding that a '*child centred approach means keeping the child in focus when making decisions about their lives and working in partnership with them and their families'* (HMG, 2018, p 9). The document is central to practitioners developing both their understanding and practice. It highlights and explains the responsibility of Local Authorities in publishing how safeguarding assessments are conducted, the importance of early help, as well as making links to legislation that underpins the practice within the guidance. The guidance also highlights the need for each area to have Multi-Agency Safeguarding Arrangements (MASA). The MASA will have a website that contains all the information of your local area's response to safeguarding and will support you in this practice.

Critical questions ⑦

After exploring the contemporary landscape of safeguarding, consider the following questions.

» Have you read the Working together to safeguard children (2018) guidance? Take some time to do this. Note down significant practice points and discuss these with your safeguarding lead with the workplace.

» Are you aware of your local MASA? If not research this by exploring your local MASA website.

Stories of practice need to be authentic and honest to have value in making use of the experiences of others. We need to be real about the emotions at play throughout our practice. The case study below will support you in reflecting on some of the potential emotions stirred by thinking about or enacting the riskier aspects of practice and how to support yourself in becoming courageous in our work with children and families. Writing this case study has been part of my journey in finding and becoming confident in my own voice (see Chapter 1) and in validating the emotions I was previously ashamed of to bolster my practice. I hope that it will provide the same validation for you so that you can lean into the humanness of your professional identity and support your professional self in a way that is meaningful.

CASE STUDY ⤶

Emma's story

Emma began her BA (Hons) Early Childhood in 2014 as a mature student, full-time childminder and mother of two. In 2017 she continued into a MA Education with an early years specialism, before beginning her teacher training with Teach First in 2019 – by this point with four children. Her story describes some of the hurdles she experienced along the way.

I was a 'mature' student when I embarked upon the Early Childhood Professional Practice degree. At 22, I had two children and had worked in childcare since leaving school. More than anything, I had hoped the degree would bring a depth of conversation around my practice and I arrogantly assumed I would be one of the more confident students given my experience. To some extent this was the case. At times, however, I was not bolstered by my practice experience but instead crushed by it. In my second year, one of the year-long modules was on safeguarding and while I knew this was crucial to my practice and was grateful for the opportunity to understand it better, I found my overall takeaway from most lectures was abject terror. If I'm honest, before studying this module, rather than reflect about safeguarding issues my instinct was to avoid thinking about them at all costs and hope I never had to put training into practice. Accepting the weight of the responsibility I had to the children in my care, and really considering the ways in which children have fallen through the gaps in the past paralysed me and no amount of policy or training seemed to help. Simultaneously, however, I realised the impact that this fear of safeguarding issues could have on my willingness to recognise and act upon them in practice. I desperately sought some equilibrium in my conception of safeguarding in practice. When the time came to move back into practice, I found that my fear of this issue meant that I immediately sought secure knowledge of the specifics of safeguarding policy in school and most crucially, 'who do I go to for help?'. This served as an emotional anchor for me regarding my fears and meant that I felt less isolated in my responsibility and more capable of action. Alongside this, it was important to re-conceptualise those who 'need to know' as an opportunity to engage an appropriate agent to help me support children further as opposed to being an exclusively limiting factor in seeking help.

My teacher training year challenged my relationship with policy in this regard, as it coincided with the emergence of the Covid-19 pandemic and the disruption to schools that followed. As a qualified first-aider, I was signposted as one of the points of contact in case of positive symptoms of Covid-19. I found this evoked that familiar terror I had come to associate with the safeguarding aspect of my role, and it was at this point that I came to recognise the usual places I sought comfort in the face of fear, people and policy. This time was different though. There was no precedence for this, and no policy which existed in responding to it. Without these anchors I felt more at sea than ever. Having spoken to other first-aiders, I found that this was a shared feeling and that we felt unprepared in our role, again just hoping we would never have to enact the role in practice. However, given the universal lack of certainty about how to handle the emerging Covid-19 situation and therefore my inability to seek guidance in school, I knew this was an unsustainable position that needed to be addressed. In order to tackle this, I decided to create the policy I needed. Using the whole-school risk assessment as a basis, and with the permission of senior leadership, I developed policy for the staff handbook which described the procedure should someone display positive Covid-19 symptoms. While this was with the purpose of understanding better my role in this context, a more long-term learning point for me was the emotional safety required for practitioners to act effectively in difficult circumstances and the potential role of policy in supporting this. This was the first time I felt that policy was supportive of my practice rather than being an expectation to meet and, as such, was truly purposeful. Creating this policy allowed me to feel more comfortable in the aspects of my practice that keep others safe than I had experienced before and gave me vastly more confidence in my practice than an awareness of policy ever has.

Critical questions ⑦

»   Do you recognise any of these emotions within your own practice?

»   What could the impact of fear be if it were to go unchecked?

»   Where does Emma usually seek safety in these situations? Where can you go to address any fears you might have?

»   Who has created the policies within your placement setting?

»   Within this case study, what was the impact of the creation of policy that is responsive to the needs of the setting and the people within it?

»   What could the impact be if staff feel emotionally safe and confident about their practice?

Keeping yourself safe: developing your personalised toolkit

It is important to consider what constitutes a safe place to work. Emma's case study highlights that safety is not just about avoiding accidents or physical harm but is indicative also of an interactive relationship between a person and the multiple elements of their environment. How the environment interacts with the person's feelings, what it expects of the person and how it supports them in achieving this all play a role in the sense of safety experienced. This suggests that what is required to keep a person safe is idiosyncratic and unique to each of us. To illustrate this, it is worth exploring what safety might mean to some of the different people in setting. An adaptation of Brookfield's (2017) lenses provides a useful frame through which to view this (see also Chapter 2).

Figure 6.1 shows the factors which may attribute to a feeling of safety for different people within a setting. It highlights that for children, safety might be about whether their friends want to play with them, whereas for an adult it could be about how safe their job feels. It is important to acknowledge that the perceived answers to these questions are dynamic in response to the emerging needs of the individual and the interactions they have in setting on any given day. It is also important to recognise the reductive nature of this illustration and that not all children will be concerned with the same things. For example, the child who has experienced trauma in early life might be more concerned with sudden loud noises than the child who was once bitten by a dog (see Chapter 7). The autobiographical lens is an opportunity to decide for yourself what safety looks like in a setting. Emma's case study highlights the potential for our fears to become shadows on our practice. Shadows we actively avoid considering because reflecting on these fears can be uncomfortable. It also highlights, however, the courage and empowerment that can be cultivated by leaning into this discomfort,

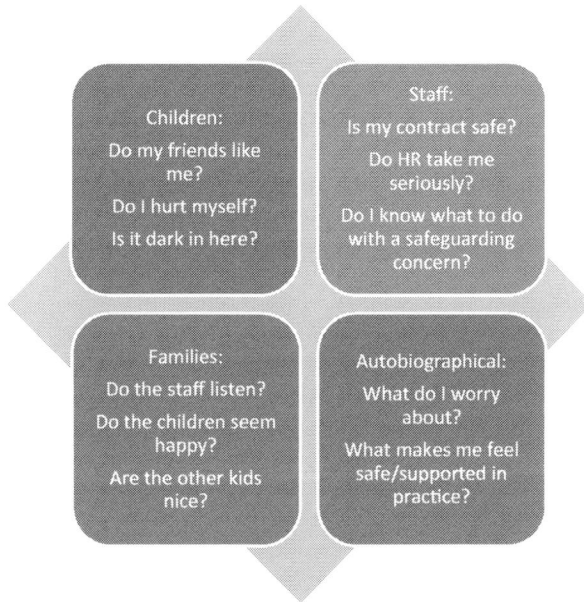

Figure 6.1 *How safe do I feel model, adapted from Brookfield's (2017) lenses*

shining a light on those fears and considering them carefully and systematically as an area worthy of reflection.

A useful time to begin creating your own personal toolkit is just before placement experiences (see Chapter 3). Understandably, many students feel a great deal of nerves prior to embarking on a new placement opportunity but this is a valuable opportunity for reflection that can support your practice before you even arrive. Whether you already have gained practice experience or are about to, consider the feelings you have in the weeks and days running up to this; take time to think about '*what feelings are you experiencing?*' and '*what are you most excited about?*' and '*what makes you most nervous?*' Your responses to these questions will produce valuable insight about yourself and your practice and serve as a sort of sub-conscious risk assessment that we may often fail to confront or avoid.

Reflection on Emma's story

Below are some questions which will support you in understanding better the very human needs that also form part of your individual and professional identity. By answering these questions as honestly as possible, you can begin to piece together a picture of what you need within your professional environment to feel confident in your practice. This activity contributes to building a toolkit in supporting you and your practice.

Time to consider 💭

»   Consider your answers to the autobiographical questions contained in Figure 6.1 and what this lens might look like for you. What sort of questions would you ask of your setting in order to feel safe? These might reflect the sort of worries you might feel on a Sunday night when considering the week ahead or the parts of your day that you ruminate on while you drive home.

»   Organise these questions under the titles; 'Physical', 'Emotional' and 'Social' well-being and consider each of these areas as fully as possible.

»   If you notice any specific fears you have or areas of practice that make you uncomfortable, then try and articulate these as specifically as you can. What is your fear? What would happen if this came true? What would the impact be on you? What would the impact be on others (your colleagues/the children/their families)? How would this make you feel?

»   What resources are available to you? Who can help you? Are there policies that exist already or could be put in place to strengthen your approach in this area of practice? Does further training exist? Do others feel the way that you do?

»   Looking again at the lenses above (including your autobiographical lens), how could you support a sense of safety of others in setting?

Chapter summary 📖

This chapter has explored our duties in safeguarding the welfare of the children we work with. Having explored the legislative landscape of safeguarding, it was important to take an honest look at the emotions that may be stirred by what can feel like a risky element of our practice. We then looked at some of the tools available to us in order to support ourselves both personally and professionally. This is crucial in building the courage required to work with children and families.

Further reading 📖

Department for Education (DfE) (2021) *Keeping Children Safe in Education*. London: HMSO.

• This document gives the latest guidance and is worth reading if you are working in education.

Frost, N (2021) *Safeguarding Children and Young People: A Guide for Professionals Working Together*. London: Sage.

• This newly published book explores recent changes in policy and practice as well as offering good practice suggestions and approaches.

Walker, G (2018) *Working Together for Children. A Critical Introduction to Multi-agency Working.* London: Bloomsbury.

• This book is a firm favourite with students. It is written in an accessible way that helps to support a critical approach within your reading.

References ⬥

Brookfield, S (2017) *Becoming a Critically Reflective Teacher* (2nd ed). New Jersey: Jossey-Bass.

Cruelty to Animals Act (1876). [online] Available at: www.legislation.gov.uk/ukpga/Vict/39-40/77/enacted (accessed 20 January 2022).

Department for Education (DfE) (2011) *The Munro Review of Child Protection Final Report.* London: HMSO. [online] Available at: www.gov.uk/government/publications/munro-review-of-child-protection-final-report-a-child-centred-system (accessed 9 November 2021).

Department for Education (DfE) (2021) *Keeping Children Safe in Education 2021.* London: HMSO. [online] Available at: https://assets.publishing.service.gov.uk/government/uploads/system/uploads/attachment_data/file/1021914/KCSIE_2021_September_guidance.pdf (accessed 9 November 2021).

Department for Education and Skills (DfES) (2003) *Every Child Matters.* London: HMSO. [online] Available at: https://assets.publishing.service.gov.uk/government/uploads/system/uploads/attachment_data/file/272064/5860.pdf (accessed 9 November 2021).

Frost, N (2021) *Safeguarding Children and Young People: A Guide for Professionals Working Together.* London: Sage.

Gallagher, S and Sutton-Tsang, S (2017) Safeguarding: Understanding Your Responsibilities. In Musgrave, J, Savin-Badin, M and Stobbs, N (eds) *Studying for Your Early Years Degree: Skills and Knowledge for Becoming an Effective Practitioner.* St Albans: Critical Publishing.

HM Government (2016) *Wood Report Review of the Role and Functions of Local Safeguarding Children Boards.* London: HMSO. [online] Available at: www.gov.uk/government/publications/wood-review-of-local-safeguarding-children-boards (accessed 9 November 2021).

HM Government (2018) *Working Together to Safeguard Children.* London: HMSO. [online] Available at: https://assets.publishing.service.gov.uk/government/uploads/system/uploads/attachment_data/file/942454/Working_together_to_safeguard_children_inter_agency_guidance.pdf (accessed 9 November 2021).

Laming, H (2003) *The Victoria Climbie Inquiry: Report of an Inquiry by Lord Laming.* London: HMSO. [online] Available at: www.gov.uk/government/publications/the-victoria-climbie-inquiry-report-of-an-inquiry-by-lord-laming (accessed 9 November 2021).

Myers, J (2004) *A History of Child Protection in America.* Philadelphia, PA: Xlibris.

Powell, J and Uppal, E (2012). *Safeguarding Babies and Young Children: A Guide for Early Years Professionals.* New York: McGraw-Hill.

Prevention of Cruelty to, and Protection of, Children Act (1889). [online] Available at: www.legislation.gov.uk/ukpga/1889/44/enacted (accessed 9 November 2021).

7 Understanding and responding to adverse childhood experiences in practice

ERICA STRUDLEY-BROWN AND ALISON PROWLE

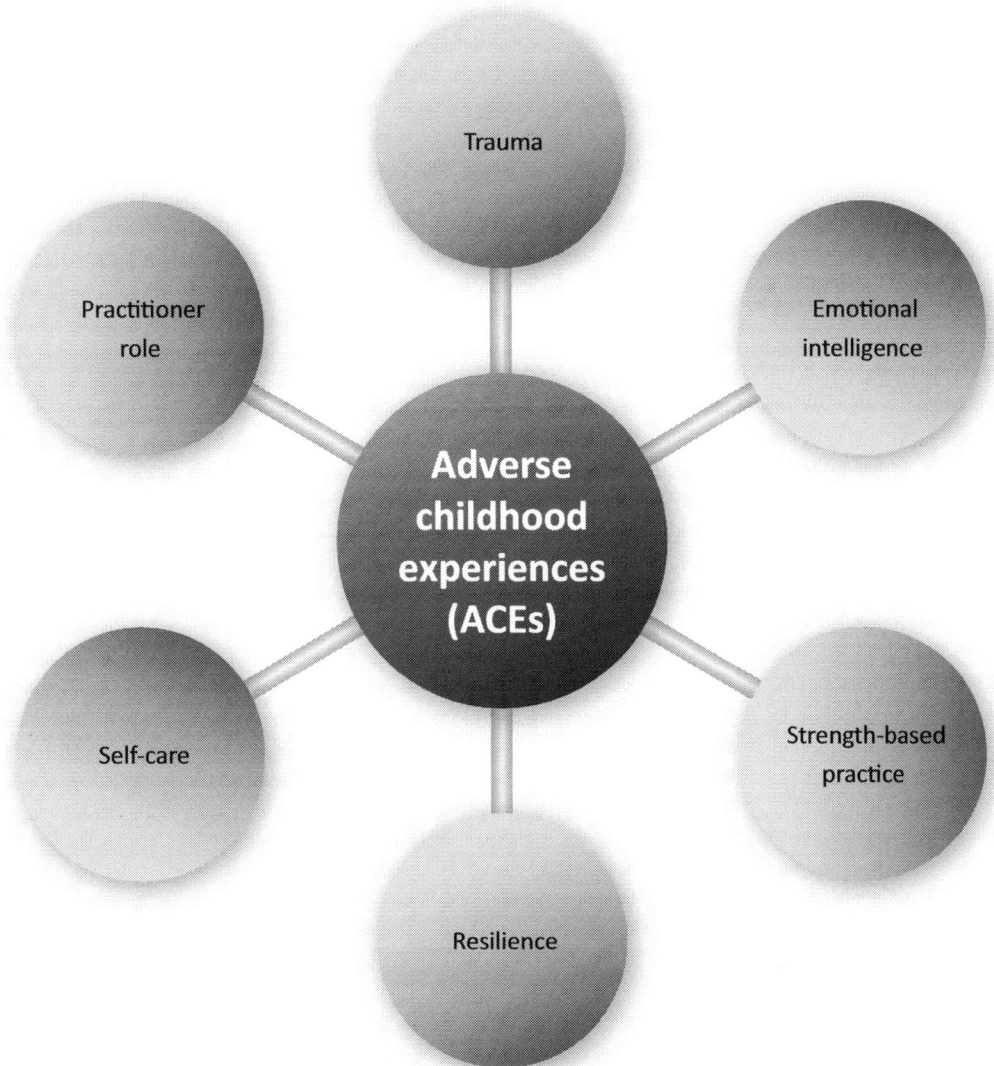

Trauma

Emotional intelligence

Practitioner role

Adverse childhood experiences (ACEs)

Self-care

Strength-based practice

Resilience

Chapter objectives ◎

This chapter aims to help those that work with children and their families to reflect on children's understanding of adverse life events and their responses to these events. It will also support practitioners in exploring their professional responsibility to care for their own well-being. Throughout the chapter, the voices of real children are used to provide a powerful insight into their lived experience and enhance our understanding. This chapter:

- explores practical ways of supporting children;

- adopts a strength-based and solution-focused approach;

- considers your own life experience and training and opportunities to develop strategies for interacting with children and their families so that you meet their individual needs and help them develop resilience;

- supports you in developing your own setting's statement of purpose as a blueprint for developing its ethos in practice.

Introduction

Within numerous studies, Adverse Childhood Experiences (ACEs) have been found to have life-long impacts on health, well-being and behaviour (eg Chapman et al, 2004; Bellis et al, 2014). It is important to recognise at the start of this chapter that some students may themselves have experienced adversity, and to consider how they may be affected when encountering children in practice who may be experiencing similar challenges. This chapter therefore starts with an author reflection to introduce some of the thinking and experiences it will consider.

CASE STUDY

Author reflection – Erica

The classroom door burst open, and two 6-year-olds rushed up to where I was preparing for the afternoon creativity lesson. 'Jessica's dad got squashed by the dustbin lorry. He's dead and her gran is coming to tell you.' I barely had time to respond to what I had been told before two huddled figures joined the three of us in the corner of the classroom. I asked the two messengers to return to the playground and searched helplessly in the depths of my mind for something my teacher training must have taught me about the situation before me. I didn't find the answer then, nor in the remainder of that first year of Qualified Teacher Status. Fifty years later, faced with the same scenario, I am sure that I would still feel ill-equipped, though at least now I have 50 years' experience to draw on.

Within all our lives there are changes and associated losses which are necessary aspects of growth and change (eg the transition to a new school), but there are also losses that do not happen to everyone. These are sometimes called 'circumstantial' losses and include situations like family breakdown, homelessness, the death of a family member or a friend, abuse, the imprisonment of a family member, and serious illness or injury. Such losses can be considered ACEs which could be defined as: '*highly stressful, and potentially traumatic, events or situations that occur during childhood and/or adolescence. They can be a single event, or prolonged threats to, and breaches of, the young person's safety, security, trust or bodily integrity*' (Brennan et al, 2019). Such adverse experiences can have both immediate and long-term consequences for children. Perhaps the most damaging effects are those which are harmful to mother–child relationships, but ACEs may also impact physical, social and emotional outcomes. Despite this, children's adverse life experiences are not directly addressed in curriculum guidelines and children continue to be assessed against national norms, ignoring the impact adverse life circumstances may have on their holistic well-being and learning. The opening sentence of Leo Tolstoy's (1878) novel *Anna Karenina* rings unquestionably true for many children. He writes, '*All happy families are alike; each unhappy family is unhappy in its own way*'. In other words, happy families share a common set of attributes that lead to happiness, while a whole variety of attributes can cause an unhappy family. Recognising the uniqueness of families and developing a robust understanding of ACEs can help your setting to proactively support families.

Time to consider 💭

» What are your setting's aims (statement of purpose)?

» How are these lived out in the opportunities given to children?

» What mechanisms are in place to support children and families with adverse life experiences?

» What is in place to support staff (and students)?

Theory and literature

Managing adverse life experiences: Erikson's psychosocial theory

The American psychologist and psychoanalyst Erikson (1963) proposed a theory that attempted to define social maturation as an eight-stage model of psychosocial development spanning infancy to adulthood. According to Erikson, each child's development follows the same stages, though individual children experience varying (positive or negative) events during each phase of their development, and a child experiencing negative setbacks is likely to have unresolved crises in later life. The first 4 of Erikson's stages, which are relevant to early childhood, are illustrated in Figure 7.1.

Stage	Age	Name	Crisis	Focus
1	0–1	*Infancy*	trust vs mistrust	mother
2	2–3	*Toddler*	autonomy vs shame	parents
3	4–5	*Pre-school*	initiative vs guilt	family
4	6–12	*Childhood*	industry vs inferiority	school, friends, home

Figure 7.1 *The first four of Erikson's psychosocial development stages (adapted from Erikson, 1963)*

According to Erikson (1963), there are four early stages of psychosocial development.

1. Infancy (0–1 year): the infant develops *trust* or *mistrust* in themselves and others. The attachment figure (mother, or another primary carer) is central.

2. Toddler (2–3 years): the child develops *autonomy* or *shame (doubt),* becoming either more independent or developing shame and doubt. Parents and significant carers are central at this stage.

3. Pre-school (4–5 years): the child shows *initiative (curiosity)* or *guilt* and endeavours to discover what sort of person they are. The extended family is significant at this point.

4. Childhood (6–12 years): the child is *industrious* or feels *inferior* at home, school and with contacts in the wider community.

Emotional intelligence and emotional literacy theory

Research around emotional intelligence and emotional literacy suggests they contribute to better health, higher academic achievement and stronger relationships (Rupande, 2015). The terms 'emotional intelligence' and 'emotional literacy' both refer to the ability to recognise, understand, handle and appropriately express emotions. 'Emotional intelligence' is a person's overall ability to deal with their emotions, while 'emotional literacy' suggests a person's ability to communicate their emotions through words and read them in others.

There are five main aspects of emotional intelligence that, when developed, lead to children becoming emotionally literate. These are identified by Goleman (1996, 2004):

• **knowing emotions** – a child recognises a feeling as it happens;

• **managing emotions** – a child has ways of reassuring themselves when they feel anxious or upset;

• **self-motivation** – a child is aware of their emotions and owns their emotions, rather than being controlled by them;

- **empathy** – a child is aware of what another person is feeling;

- **handling relationships** – a child is confident to form relationships with others.

Some children are instinctively in tune with their feelings and emotions, and they will be readily able to cope with new situations and new people. Others may need more help; hence, the impact of ACEs will vary. However, all children need to have their emotional literacy nurtured, supported and encouraged. Helping children express themselves appropriately empowers them to navigate situations as they grow up in a fast-changing world.

Critical questions ⑦

» How does your practice encourage children to develop emotional intelligence?

» What resources or approaches could you use to support children to develop emotional intelligence?

The effect of trauma

Traumatic events strike unexpectedly, turning everyday experiences upside down. They destroy the belief that '*it could never happen to me*'. The impact of any event which is unexpected, recent, or otherwise, is as horrific as it appears to the child at the time and in the days and weeks that follow. This response will be highly individual and therefore it is important that the practitioner does not make assumptions about what constitutes a 'normal' response.

While trauma is a human response, it is also complex, incorporating a myriad of emotional, behavioural and cognitive reactions. This is particularly true for children, though little is known about young children's individual responses to such events, or why some children are more vulnerable to experiencing traumatic stress than others. Indeed, not all children will have adverse reactions to traumatic events that they have experienced directly or seen in the media. For some, reactions will be minimal or short-lived. In contrast, many are likely to experience anxiety, fear and phobias in the immediate and perhaps long term. The attuned practitioner will recognise this and work at the child's pace.

Severity

Seeing disturbing images as well as experiencing or witnessing a traumatic event can trigger a severe reaction in a child. The severity of the child's response is largely determined by the seriousness of the event itself and the duration of a child's exposure to it. This will include factors such as:

- the severity of harm or threat to the child's life or that of their loved ones;

- the suddenness of the event – such as the destruction of the child's home or a well-known building within their community;

- the degree to which the child was rendered powerless;

- whether the child was alone or with other people;
- the possibility of the event reoccurring, and the intensity and proximity of exposure to disturbing images; and
- the intensity and proximity of exposure to disturbing images.

In some cases, the nature of the event seems to determine how children respond. If the trauma involved heat, noise or darkness, children's reactions may be more intense. It is very common for children who have experienced trauma to become over or under-responsive to sensory stimuli. Their response will be highly individual, and the child may not consciously be aware of it. Developing a positive and trustful relationship with the child, observation and tuning in to their responses will help you as a practitioner to support the child appropriately.

Reaction

Although it is unlikely that children will experience all the changes in behaviour detailed in this section, many will present with observable signs of restlessness, a heightened alertness to danger and irritability or outbursts of anger and temper tantrums.

CASE STUDY ☻

Sasha

Sasha was four years old when she was woken in the middle of the night to the sound of loud banging and shouting. She got out of bed and stood at the top of the stairs, where she witnessed her father being handcuffed and escorted out of the front door by uniformed police officers. Six months later, her nursery had arranged for a local police community support officer to visit as part of a project 'People Who Help Us'. When the policewoman walked into the classroom Sasha covered her ears and screamed 'Don't take me!' Sasha was reassured by her teacher; the teacher then texted her mum who arrived immediately and sat in the class holding Sasha while the police officer talked to the other children.

Critical questions ⑦

» Research what is happening in Sasha's brain when confronted with an unexpected reminder of the original trauma.

» What support could be put in place for Sasha? (Here you might want to think not just about what can be provided within the setting, but also what may be available from other agencies).

Other common reactions include:

- panic attacks;
- regression of previously acquired skills;

- refusing to go to school or nursery;

- raised levels of anxiety;

- underachieving at school;

- separation anxiety; and

- clinging behaviour.

Reactions to traumatic events can therefore manifest themselves in different ways, with this section considering the most common. Responses to a traumatic event often emerge at night-time and impact on sleep, with many children afraid of the dark or being alone. While some struggle to get to sleep, others will wake frequently and may experience night terrors. Imagery of the event also seems to be one of the recurring effects of trauma.

CASE STUDY

Jason

Jason, aged five, was asleep the night his home caught alight. Jason recalls:

'I can smell the feeling of the house burning. My mum screamed for me. The fire engines came, and I saw everything eaten by the fire. There were big bubbles coming out the sofa like a volcano'. Four years after the event Jason still cannot tolerate the smell of toast cooking, the sound of a fire engine siren or media coverage of fires.

Many children will experience a phase of denial and numbing. After this, a child may be confronted with intrusive, repetitive recollections of the event.

CASE STUDY

Rory

Rory, aged three, was on a camping holiday by the sea with his family. One night a spring tide battered the sea wall at the bottom of the campsite causing local damage and washing away beach huts. For the remainder of the holiday Rory insisted on sleeping with his parents 'in case the water comes to get us'.

Children need to make sense of their experiences and so will search for meaning to understand both the traumatic event and their feelings. Many children who have been the victims of trauma believe they were in some way responsible for what happened. Thus, a child who has witnessed a violent attack either in their home or in the environment may believe their behaviour contributed to the event. Others may be confused about why they are frightened, especially if they see other people apparently unaffected. Adults need to be open and honest and admit that sometimes there is no rational explanation for what happened. Very young children may not have the language to describe how they feel and may battle with the intensity of their emotions. They may never have experienced intense emotions before, and it is not unusual for them to attempt to repress these unknown feelings. For them, the world has become unfamiliar and frightening. Below is an example of how this may be seen.

CASE STUDY ☺

Rabie

Rabie's mum had a stroke while she was driving with Rabie and her two siblings. The car went out of control and crashed into a bus. Miraculously the children were not hurt, there were no casualties among the bus passengers and Rabie's mum recovered. However, just before the crash Rabie had given her mum a sweet which she attributed to the cause of her mum's stroke. She needed constant reassurance from her family that she was not responsible for the accident. It was only when her dad asked her to share her sweets with him on a car journey that she was able to recover from the experience.

Re-experiencing the event is also a common response. Children are likely to become distressed when aspects of events remind them of their traumatic experiences. They may also relive their experiences in nightmares, flashbacks and their play, such as in role play or in their paintings and drawings.

Nurturing resilience

Healthy emotional and cognitive development is shaped by responsive interaction with adults while 'chronic' or extreme adversity can interrupt normal brain development.

CASE STUDY ☺

Twins

After seeing images on the TV of a terrorist attack, 5-year-old twin brothers asked their grandma '*Why did the bad man do it?*' Their grandma acknowledged the boys' confusion and answered as honestly as she was able, validating their concern. She told them that she didn't understand the motives of the terrorist and said, '*even grownups cannot explain*'. The boys went to school the following day and repeated what their grandma had said during a circle time activity. Several of the other children spoke about what they had seen on their televisions. The teacher encouraged the children to talk, and she organised an activity where the class drew faces that expressed emotions. At the end of the day, she met parents and explained how she had responded to the children's concerns.

Learning how to cope with adversity is an important part of healthy child development. Children who develop resilience to everyday challenges develop positive stress responses when cortisol or stress hormones are activated in the child's brain. However, when a child is exposed to repeated adversity without support, the child is likely to experience 'toxic' stress if excessive cortisol disrupts brain circuits. Toxic stress can have a cumulative toll on the child's physical and mental well-being, and research has demonstrated how early intervention is vitally important.

Many children recover from setbacks and even traumatic unexpected events and to date there is no single predictor of a healthy response to everyday challenges and traumatic events. Studies show that toddlers who have secure attachments to their primary carer and to Early Years Professionals experience minimal activation of stress hormones when frightened by an unfamiliar event (Bethel et al, 2017). However, research into the biology of stress shows how major adversity such as extreme poverty, neglect or abuse can hamper a young child's brain development and set the body's stress response on 'high alert' because safety and stability are at risk. It is important to recognise that practitioners can help children to nurture and develop resilience. A useful framework for understanding resilience and resources to support practitioners can be found on the '*Boingboing*' resilience website (Boingboing, nd) (see also Chapter 3).

Your role as a supportive adult

There appears to be no single strategy for practitioners to adopt which helps young children to develop resilience to adversity. Until the twenty-first century it was generally considered as a by-product of education or parenting, rather than a focus. Currently, it is recognised that when adults encourage children to make decisions for themselves, they encourage an internal locus of control which lays the foundation for resilience (Brown, 2019).

Supporting children involves becoming aware of the communication skills you use every day. These skills include your verbal language and your body language. The ability to communicate is central to supporting children and their families. Good communication will include understanding children's emotional responses and endeavouring to interpret whatever they are trying to tell us. Therefore, it involves your total involvement with the child so that they are in no doubt that you are doing your very best to understand how it might be to be in their shoes. However, supporting children is not just about 'doing' – it is about 'being' present and in touch with the child at their point of need. Through your supportive care, children will be helped to make sense of their life experiences. Sharing experiences helps to remove feelings of isolation and to reduce anxiety and fear. In other words, through the relationship which exists between yourself and the child, the child is enabled to 'share their story' in the knowledge that you will support them. However, when a child talks about their feelings or shares their story, they may be wondering:

- can I talk to this adult?

- will the adult listen to me?

- will the adult recognise that what I am expressing is important to me?

- can I trust this adult?

Practitioners working with children and their families can use basic counselling skills, responding to children's needs and concerns as they arise, so that together they are able to explore what is happening. Fundamental to the relationship between the child and the supportive carer is the ability of the adult to use interpersonal skills such as listening, exploring, clarifying and responding. Inevitably, however, situations will arise where practitioners will need expertise if they are to work effectively with children who have been traumatised. These skills are not learnt overnight. They are capacities gained through professional development. However, in your role as a supportive carer you will be able to perceive what the child may be experiencing and to convey this understanding sensitively and with genuine concern.

Time to consider

Think about the quality of the supportive-carer relationships you have with children.

» Does the child perceive me as giving them my full attention?

» How do I convey my empathy and understanding to the child?

» What does my verbal and non-verbal language convey to the child?

» Are my questions open-ended, inviting the child to their story?

Confidentiality and the supportive carer relationship

We all set limits in our relationships and each of us has boundaries that preserve our own identities as individuals. The strength of the boundary depends on the nature and context of the relationship. In the supportive-carer relationship between a child and an adult, the adult strives to create a safe environment where the child feels sufficiently comfortable and valued to share their experiences and concerns. For this to happen it is essential there is trust and confidentiality, but inevitably there will be times when the capacity of the adult to support the child fully will entail sharing information with other people. Therefore, it is very important to agree with the child at the beginning of the relationship that to support them fully, other people may need to be involved.

A helpful model for managing boundaries can be found in the social pedagogy concept of the 3Ps: namely, professional, personal and private selves. As practitioners, we seek to interact in ways that are professional but also personal, keeping private those aspects that we do not want to share or that may not be beneficial to the people we support (Thempra Social Pedagogy CIC, 2019). This protects both us and the people we are working with, avoiding inappropriate disclosure which can leave both parties vulnerable. There may, of course, be times when it is appropriate to share your own experiences, but this needs to be carefully considered and reflected upon with a view to keeping everyone safe.

All settings will have policies which relate to safeguarding and teachers should be clear on how to respond if a child shares personal information or something comes to their attention that may affect either their short-term or long-term welfare. We can also reassure children that:

- we will not reveal information carelessly or unnecessarily;

- any information they share will only be discussed with people who need to know, and that other people will treat the information confidentially;

- their welfare is of prime importance;

- if it is necessary to share information with other people you will ask the child's permission to do this.

Using counselling and communication skills

When children are unhappy, they often find it hard to concentrate which may mean that in conversations which they have with us they are darting around from one subject to another. Although this may be helpful to the child because it gives them autonomy to choose what they say, it can be very difficult to gain a clear picture of what is happening. Taking time during the conversation to summarise what the child has said so far may have two helpful outcomes. First, it helps the child to know that what they have said is important and second it helps the adult to check that they have understood correctly. Summarising does not mean just a mechanical repetition, however. It means finding our own words to reflect to the child what they have said, both in content and in the emotions they have expressed.

Having feelings understood can be very affirming. To be fully in touch with how children express emotions, we need to listen very carefully to what they say and how their levels of emotional response are articulated. There will be times when children who are usually verbally articulate will be at a loss for words. This is especially so when they are struggling with painful feelings. Silence may seem prolonged and uncomfortable for the adult but generally it is not like this for the child. Space for thought may give them an opportunity to reflect on what is happening to them and to communicate this in a different way, for example, through their body language or play.

There is a special quality about reflective silence which embraces an acceptance and understanding. Therefore, it is important not to interrupt too soon. The child may be supported non-verbally through gesture or perhaps through holding their hand. There will also be occasions when empathetic listening will involve talking to the child about what we suspect is troubling them, enabling them to explore their own thoughts and experiences. Direct and indirect questions may also be helpful. In summary the child needs an adult who:

- conveys empathy;

- is non-judgmental and does not show a shocked reaction to anything shared;

- allows them to express their emotions;

- checks they understand what has been communicated;

- uses open-ended questions;

- helps them to make sense of their experiences;

- they can trust;

- offers a safe environment.

Caring for colleagues and ourselves

When working with children and their families caring extends beyond the child who has experienced adversity. The child is part of their home, family and a member of the setting family, so in reaching out to the child, you may also find yourself caring for the needs of the parents, the child's peer group, the family, colleagues and yourself. Although not all families need professional intervention, many will welcome support. Practitioners have a responsibility to reach out to families and to communicate their willingness to offer support and guidance.

Caring for each other

Practitioners may experience stress as a result of a commitment to caring for others (see Chapter 5). Often this effects the carer's personal life. Peer support is very important since carers need opportunities to interact with colleagues in equal two-way relationships.

Caring will involve:

- an awareness of how colleagues respond to stress;

- acknowledging the stress colleagues are under;

- encouraging colleagues to seek specialist professional support if necessary;

- a willingness to offer support.

In effective settings, people have time for each other amidst the hustle and bustle of activity. Nevertheless, some people are more comfortable supporting colleagues than others. Sharing responsibilities with colleagues provides an opportunity for continuity of care as well as protection from stress and burnout. Team relationships are important (see Chapter 8). In many ways they involve the same principles as working with children and their families. There are two fundamental capacities associated with the role of caring for others – effective communication and an awareness and interest in interacting with other people. Where practitioners are successfully supported by other people their needs are respected. This respect will be affirmed through:

- helping each other to feel at ease;

- creating an atmosphere that is relaxed yet purposeful;

- giving each other individual attention;

- safeguarding against distractions when we are attending to others' needs;

- contributing helpful resources.

It is important to recognise that practitioners may find situations that arise upsetting (see Chapter 6). Where strong team relationships exist, colleagues can provide support in these circumstances. However, sometimes, it may not feel that support is available. Supervision and support from managers are critical in allowing for a reflective unpacking of situations, emotions, interventions and solutions (see also Chapter 9). For students, your personal academic tutor may also be able to provide support and signpost to other sources of help and information.

Caring for ourselves

The relationship which exists between the practitioners and a child or his or her family is often an asymmetric one where we do most of the giving and the child and the family do a large proportion of the receiving. It is important that we can recognise our own emotional depletion. This will include:

* feeling overworked and unable to delegate;

* feeling physically exhausted and ineffective;

* feeling hopeless and helpless;

* low motivation;

* physical illness and vulnerability to infection;

* negative attitudes towards other people; and

* gaining little job satisfaction.

Our willingness to support families should not undermine our own needs. It is important to ensure that our own well-being needs are addressed, from the basics of sleep, good nutrition and exercise through to finding time to connect with others and take part in activities we enjoy (Prowle and Hodgkins, 2020) (see also Chapter 3). We also need to recognise that our own life experiences may impact on our ability to support children and families in adverse circumstances. The following case study explores how supporting children and families in adversity may generate difficult feelings for the practitioner.

CASE STUDY ↪

Andrea, childhood studies placement student, Year 1

As part of the second year of her degree programme Andrea was required to undertake a three-week placement in a Year 1 class. Andrea was quickly able to establish a rapport with the children and found that some of the children really enjoyed their one-to-one time with her while she was listening to them read. One of the children, Amelia, shared with her that her dad had recently moved out of the family home, and she now saw him twice a week.

→

Amelia was clearly bewildered by the situation and was very keen to talk about why this had happened. She was very tearful and found it hard to settle down to reading. Andrea made sure that the classteacher was told about the conversation but later that evening, she found herself getting very upset.

Andrea's own father had died suddenly when she was seven. She found herself thinking back to the funeral and the weeks that followed it. She vividly remembered feeling like she had to be brave for her mum and baby brother. As she sat now in her student flat, she felt very overwhelmed and had physical symptoms of nausea and lightheadedness. Andrea felt that she did not want to go back to the placement and began to worry that she would never realise her dream of becoming a teacher.

Critical questions ⑦

» Can you draw upon any theory to help understand the situation Andrea finds herself in?

» How could the classteacher and/or her personal academic tutor best support Andrea? What other support may be available?

» What strategies could Andrea herself use to help her manage the situation?

Chapter summary 📖

Because we are all different, the ways in which we react in the face of adversity and the coping strategies which we adopt will be unique to each of us. How well a child copes with a traumatic experience is dependent on several interrelating factors – the child's own cognitive ability and capacity to express their emotions, and the level of stability and support that they enjoy within and outside the home, including the presence of primary carers and significant others in the child's life and familiar routines.

There will be areas where your skills exceed ours as the authors of this chapter. There will be other areas where you can learn from others around you. It is important that you keep developing your 'toolbox' for supporting children and families, while recognising the following points.

• There is no single way to support children and families. Yet there are avenues open to each one of us.

• Keep travelling alongside people whatever their age, listen to the words they use to express their experiences and the ways they choose to communicate with you.

• Place yourself with the child and their family and be sensitive to their need to be active participants in what is happening to them.

- Give your support but do not lose sight of the emotional price which you pay for your own commitment.

- Seek solace, guidance and comfort for yourself. But most importantly trust the children and their families to be your guide.

Further reading

Brown, E (2018) *Life Changes 2: Loss, Change and Bereavement for Young People Aged 11–16 Years*. Manchester: Lions International.

• A valuable resource that has been used in schools, for example in the aftermath of the Grenfell Tower disaster.

Burke Harris, N (2014) How Childhood Trauma Affects Health Across a Lifetime. TedMed. [online] www.ted.com/talks/nadine_burke_harris_how_childhood_trauma_affects_health_across_a_ lifetime?langugage=eng (accessed 15 March 2022, run time approx 16 minutes)

• Paediatrician Nadine Burke Harris explains that the repeated stress of abuse, neglect and parents struggling with mental health or substance abuse issues has real, tangible effects on the development of the brain.

Boingboing (undated) www.boingboing.org

• This very helpful website includes a myriad of resources to support practitioners in promoting children's resilience. There are thought-provoking articles, useful activities and up-to-date research. The website also includes a helpful resilience framework: Resilience Framework *(Children and Young People) 2012 – Boingboing, adapted from Hart and Blincow with Thomas 2007.*

References

Bellis, M A, Hughes, K, Leckenby, N, Perkins, C and Lowey, H (2014) National Household Survey of Adverse Childhood Experiences and Their Relationship with Resilience to Health-harming Behaviours in England. *BMC Medicine*, 12(72). [online] Available at: https://bmcmedicine.biomed central.com/articles/10.1186/1741-7015-12-72#citeas (accessed 6 December 2019).

Bethell, C, Carle, A, Hudziak, J, Gombojav, N, Powers, K, Wade, R and Braveman, P (2017) Methods to Assess Adverse Childhood Experiences of Children and Families: Toward Approaches to Promote Child Well-being in Policy and Practice. *Academic Paediatrics*, 17(7): S51–S69.

Brown, E (2019) *Life Changes: Loss, Change and Bereavement for Children Aged 3–11 Years Old*. Manchester: Lions Clubs UK.

Cherniss, C (2000) *Emotional Intelligence; What Is It and Why Does It Matter?* Consortium for Research on Emotional Intelligence in Organizations. [online] Available at: www.researchgate.net/ publication/228359323_Emotional_intelligence_What_it_is_and_why_it_matters (accessed 20 January 2022).

Dyregrov, A (2008) *Grief in Children: A Handbook for Adults* (2nd ed). London: Jessica Kingsley.

Erikson, E H (1963) *Childhood and Society* (2nd ed). New York: W W Norton & Company.

Goleman, D (1996) Emotional Intelligence. Why It Can Matter more than IQ. *Learning*, 24(6): 49–50.

Goleman, D (2004) *Working with Emotional Intelligence*. London: Bloomsbury Press.

Hauser, M (2021) How Early Life Adversity Transforms the Learning Brain. *Mind, Brain and Education*, 15(1): 35–47.

Heard-Garris, N, Davis, M M, Szilagyi, M and Kan, K (2018) Childhood Adversity and Parent Perceptions of Child Resilience. *BMC Paediatrics*, 18(1): 1–10.

Lewis, R (2020) *Erikson's 8 Stages of Psychosocial Development Explained to Parents*. [online] Available at: www.healthline.com/health/parenting/erikson-stages (accessed 2 August 2021).

Mooney, C G (2013) *Theories of Childhood: An Introduction to Dewey, Montessorri, Erikson, Piaget and Vygotsky*. San Paul: Redleaf Press.

Prowle, A and Hodgkins, A (2021) *Making a Difference with Children and Families; Re-imagining the Role of the Practitioner*. London: Macmillan.

Rupande, G (2015) Institutionalized Discrimination in the Education System and Beyond: Themes and Perspectives. *International Journal of Humanities Social Sciences and Education (IJHSSE)*, 2(1): 245–55.

Santos, R, Fettig, A and Shafter, L (2012) Helping Families Connect: Early Literacy with Social-Emotional Development. *Young Children,* 67(2): 88–93.

ThemPra Social Pedagogy CIC (2019) *Key Concepts in Social Psychology*. [online] Available at: www.thempra.org.uk/social-pedagogy/ (accessed 15 September 2021).

Tolstoy, L (2014 [1878]) *Anna Karenina*. Surrey: Alma Classics.

8 Developing workplace relationships

SAMANTHA SUTTON-TSANG

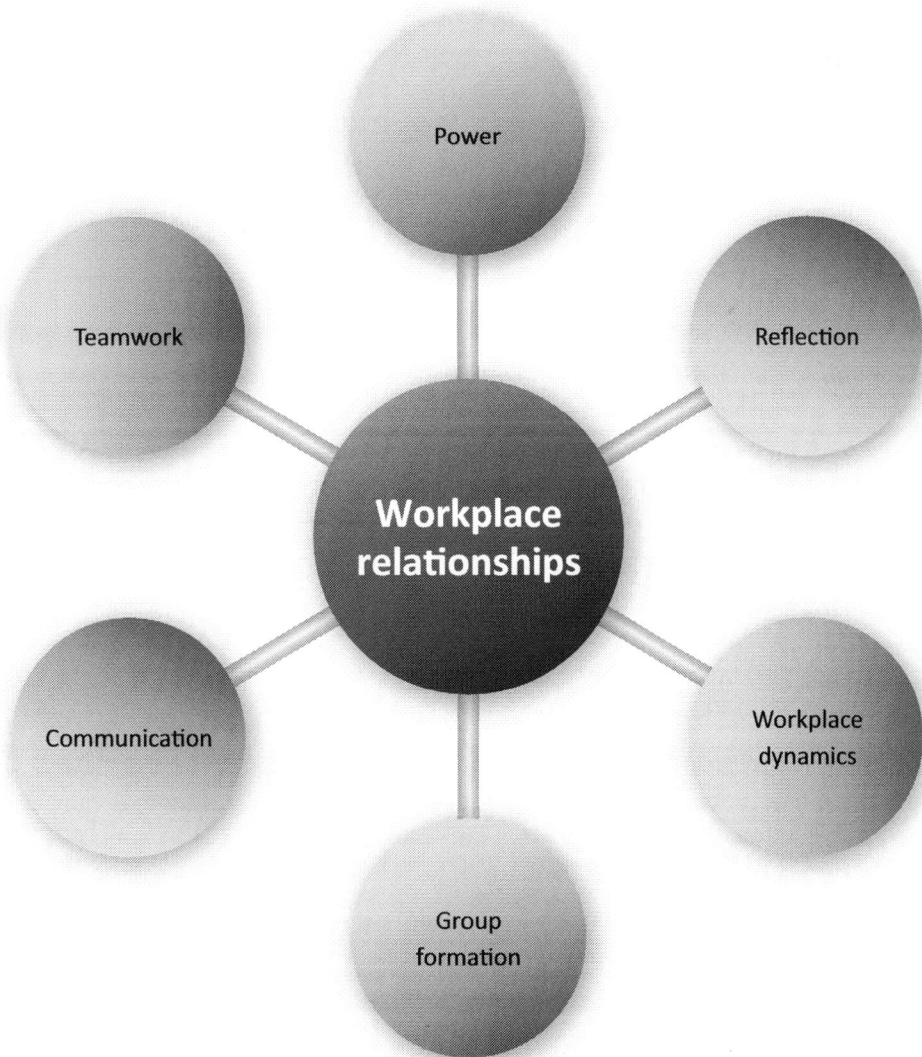

Chapter objectives ◎

This chapter explores the relationships and power struggles that practitioners and students can sometimes face within the workplace. This chapter:

- enables you to reflect on your experience of working with others;

- explores theory related to effective teamwork;

- considers the experiences of working with others using a case study example;

- uses critical questions to support you to identify key challenges, responses and solutions when developing workplace relationships.

Introduction

This chapter provides guidance to students starting out in placement and for practitioners working with children and families who may be transitioning to a new status within an organisation (see Chapter 10). It also supports and enables you to reflect on how to develop healthy balanced workplace relationships even if you have worked in a setting for some time.

Although having a new challenge can be exciting, starting a new job or placement can be stressful. Learning new policies, procedures and routines, and getting to know the staff team and children are some of the pressures involved when starting a new role or setting.

This chapter considers workplace relations. Where positive relationships exist, practitioners will be supported, and challenged, to progress their skills and horizons (see Chapter 1). In contrast, some workplace relationships may be negative, in that they are critical and can undermine confidence and practice. This leads to practitioners being disempowered rather than being empowered and strengthened, and potentially a toxic work environment.

Harder, Wagner and Rash (2014, p 207) apply Appelbaum and Roy-Girard's (2007) research on '*Toxins in the workplace*' and define a toxic work environment as '*Environments that negatively impact the long-term viability of an organization ... [which] can be considered toxic if it is ineffective as well as destructive to its employees*'. Later in this chapter, we explore an example of this as part of Carrie's case study to demonstrate how the work environment can impact on an individual's level of anxiety.

So, what can you do to transition into a setting and develop positive workplace relationships? One way is to gain an understanding of how power relationships and team dynamics work, as this can help you identify your place within an already established organisation as well as identifying where and how you can thrive.

Power

The Oxford Dictionary defines 'power' as the capacity or ability to direct or influence the behaviour of others or the course of events, whereas 'power dynamics' describes how power affects a relationship between two or more people. This can be applied to 'organisation power' where one individual has the potential to exhibit power over another (Martinez et al, 2012). While Martinez et al (2012) focus on leader-member power exchanges, the focus of this chapter is on the effect that power has within workplace relationships. Power dynamics and relationships are discussed further in several publications including Emerson (1962) and Pfeffer (1992). Emerson (1962) provides a theory on power-dependence relations based on his research into four types of balancing operations; Pfeffer (1992) addresses the complexities of organisational power and balance and clarifies the skills necessary to understand and use it in practice effectively.

French and Raven (1959) conducted a study that theorised that five main types of power exist.

1. **Coercive power**: the ability to offer punishments to deter certain actions. For example, the police can arrest law breakers; therefore, the public should adhere to laws enforced.

2. **Reward power**: the ability to give out rewards for desired behaviour. For example, a parent may reward their child with a treat in exchange for doing chores.

3. **Legitimate/formal power**: also known as titular power. This comes from having an official position. For example, the CEO of a company can terminate contracts of workers positioned below them in the organisational structure.

4. **Referent power**: the influence that comes from being liked by others. For example, a popular, charismatic student may create a new fashion trend at school.

5. **Expert power**: the influence that comes from having exceptional skills. For example, a talented carpenter may have a lot of power in a town that needs furniture.

(Goodtherapy.org, 2019)

In 1965, French and Bertram added two further types of power to the list.

1. **Connection power**: the ability to offer access to certain people or resources. For example, an agent can introduce an actor to a film producer.

2. **Informational power**: the influence that comes from knowledge and information. For example, a spy may know the location of an enemy base.

This list is not to say that individuals hold only one type of power at any one time, but that in different situations, multiple types of power can be adopted and may overlap. The use and effectiveness of the different types of power is situational; therefore, it is important to know when to use each power base. According to Raven (2004, p 6), 'it is of particular practical interest to know what bases of power or which power strategies are most likely to be effective, but it is clear that there is no simple answer', highlighting that there is no single formula for what works, since every situation is unique to the individual and setting.

Raven (2004) provides examples of the effectiveness of various power base combinations and the influence they have on social change. For example, if reward and coercive power bases are adopted by influencing agents, targets will comply only if they believe that the agents will be able to determine whether they complied. Another example is that a supervisor (eg manager) may adopt informational power to impart knowledge on a job role with the expectation that a subordinate (eg practitioner) will adhere to the rules, but also adopt a legitimate power base, with the subordinate understanding that if they do not perform effectively, the supervisor can terminate their contract subject to employment law.

When reflecting on the use of French and Raven's (1959) power bases in the workplace, it is possible to identify the various types of power that individual team members may have as well as your own power base to establish oneself within the workplace.

Time to consider 💭

» Reflecting on your own position in your workplace, what power bases do you hold and how could you use this to your advantage in developing team dynamics and furthering the outcomes for children and their families?

Tuckman's stages of group development

Tuckman's stages of group development is another theory that can be used to help us to understand team dynamics in an organisation. Tuckman (1965) initially identified four stages that teams progress through: forming, storming, norming and performing, to which Jensen (1977), later added the adjourning stage. Below is a brief outline of each of the stages of group development.

At each stage, communication is key. Table 8.1 also identifies strategies to support the team in moving on to the next stage. You may wish to extend this table for your own notes and to add a further column to support your reflection of practice using the second critical question below to frame your answers.

Table 8.1 An overview of Tuckman (1965) and Jensen's (1977) stages of group development

Stage	Description	Strategies to support
Forming	Team is formed, individuals get to know each other. At this initial stage, most team members are positive and polite. Some are anxious, as they haven't fully understood what work the team will do. Others are simply excited about the task ahead.	Team building activities to help build trust, build on individual's strengths and support weakness; establish expectations and clear boundaries; build a group identity and purpose.

Table 8.1 (*Cont.*)

Stage	Description	Strategies to support
Storming	Storming often starts where there is a conflict between team members' natural working styles. People may work in different ways for all sorts of reasons but, if differing working styles cause unforeseen problems, they may become frustrated. Other causes of conflict include unclear or undefined roles, responsibilities or tasks; workload overload; unsupportive workplace relationships; authority challenged; unclear team goals. It is often at this point that teams will fail.	Compromise; understand each other's strengths and weaknesses to develop mutual trust; coach behaviours that support resolution; maintain a calm working environment.
Norming	At this stage, individuals begin to resolve their differences following the Storming stage, as they start to appreciate each other's roles and efforts. It may be that the team develops a stronger relationship as they become more familiar with each other, therefore ask for help and provide constructive feedback to each other.	Revisit roles and responsibilities; check in with colleagues regularly; gather feedback from staff; recognise individual and group efforts; set aside time for planning and engaging as a team. Revisit the Forming and Storming stage if required to ensure expectations and goals are clear.
Performing	This is when all the hard work is paid off and there is a positive outcome or achievement in a goal. At the performing stage, leaders can support individual team members to develop their skills and practice further.	Model supporting behaviours; encourage continuing professional development; celebrate achievements; encourage group decision-making and problem-solving; provide opportunities to share and learn across teams.
Adjourning	Short-term project teams and even permanent teams can reach this stage when there is organisational restructure. Team members who like routine, or who have developed close working relationships with colleagues, may find this stage challenging, particularly if their future now looks uncertain. This can be an emotional stage.	Recognise and acknowledge change; allow for flexibility in team roles; provide opportunities for team evaluations; develop future leadership opportunities; provide emotional support.

Critical questions ⑦

» How does Tuckman's model resonate with your experiences from practice and teamwork?

» When working as part of a team, how could you support the team in moving through the various stages to become an effective team or to ensure a positive team dynamic?

The GRPI model

Another theory that identifies four interrelated components for effective teamwork was developed by Beckhard (1972). The GRPI (goals, roles, processes and interpersonal relationships) model can be used to identify potential causes of conflict or dysfunction in a team. Figure 8.1 outlines the four components and how these can be applied into a team or the workplace.

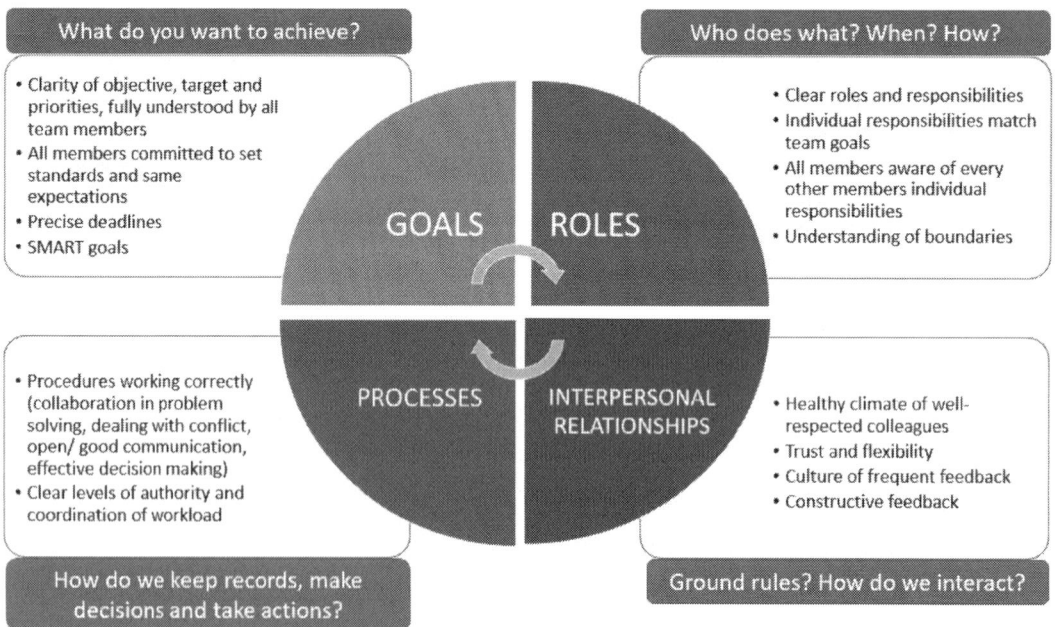

What do you want to achieve?

• Clarity of objective, target and priorities, fully understood by all team members
• All members committed to set standards and same expectations
• Precise deadlines
• SMART goals

Who does what? When? How?

• Clear roles and responsibilities
• Individual responsibilities match team goals
• All members aware of every other members individual responsibilities
• Understanding of boundaries

GOALS **ROLES**

PROCESSES **INTERPERSONAL RELATIONSHIPS**

• Procedures working correctly (collaboration in problem solving, dealing with conflict, open/ good communication, effective decision making)
• Clear levels of authority and coordination of workload

• Healthy climate of well-respected colleagues
• Trust and flexibility
• Culture of frequent feedback
• Constructive feedback

How do we keep records, make decisions and take actions?

Ground rules? How do we interact?

Figure 8.1 GRPI model for effective teamwork (adapted from Manivannan, 2020 and Accipio, 2021)

Teams can use the four question boxes (Figure 8.1) to initiate team plans, review and evaluate how well the team is working. It is useful to check in with the team, using the bullet points identified within each question to establish if individuals fully comprehend the goals of the organisation and to enable them to identify problems and propose appropriate solutions.

Now consider Carrie's reflections as an experienced primary school teacher, returning to the workplace as a teaching assistant (TA) after taking a career break to raise her children:

CASE STUDY ⊙

Carrie, teacher, reflection on returning to the workplace and integrating into a team: Part 1

After having worked seven years as a full-time classteacher in various primary schools, with many management duties, I decided to take a break to start a family. I had intended to return to teaching after a career break of one to two years at the most, but this break ended up being nine years. During that time I worked part time for my husband's business in an admin role and I enjoyed helping out at Parent Teacher Association events for my own children and also went into their school regularly as a volunteer to hear readers. I felt comfortable being on a voluntary basis due to not having the expectation to commit; volunteering was an excellent way to offer my skills and get a flavour of the workplace again, and it was welcoming and friendly.

I knew, long term, I didn't want to return to teaching full time as I wanted to be around for my own children, but I still enjoyed working with children and wanted to use some of my time and skills doing this. Having only ever been a full-time classteacher, I was hesitant to job share due to the pressures I perceived this role as having. I had seen the experience of my job share colleagues – even when talented, organised, skilled colleagues teamed up together, due to the fast paced, highly complicated nature of the job, a job share ended up being double the amount of workload, with colleagues spending as much time in preparation to handover to the other colleague as the work itself. This combined with being unable to switch off during non-teaching days, worries about curriculum overlap, gaps in planning, meeting deadlines, sometimes inevitably missing out on vital information in staff meetings, harder to make connections with TAs, other staff, parents and children due to lack of continuity.

I began to volunteer one day a week at another primary school, many of the staff I knew from my teaching days. This suited me as it was closer to home and fit around childcare. When a TA opportunity came up at the school, I applied only on the condition that I could start later and leave a little earlier in order to fit around my childcare. Many were surprised that I had decided to go for a part-time TA role but I knew it would entail less pressure with no expectation to bring work home, enabling me to carry out my other commitments. I felt it was a very gradual return to the workplace in a more formal way.

I remember being specifically asked at the interview as to why I would want a TA role and not a teaching role, and would I find it hard to adapt to working under the guidance of the teacher. I could understand how this may have had the potential to cause tension but I was clear that I knew exactly the kind of pressure a teacher is under, and therefore would be able to effectively take on some of the workloads in a supportive role. Having worked with many TAs over the years, I was clear about their role, expectations and boundaries. I felt it was useful to see how the curriculum was taught, what behaviour policies were like, and the dynamic of working with parents, the office etc. There was a good work–life balance even during the day with clearly defined break times.

→

I found the dynamic between the classteacher and I was very natural and easy as we had once worked together as teachers. I found the curriculum and planning straightforward as there were many similarities from years ago. It was great to team teach and to give the children a chance to understand their tasks. It was the classteacher who sometimes had a hard time asking me to do things like clearing up, washing up after Art, sweeping, tying shoelaces, sorting first aid, photocopying, laminating, sticking in sheets. I had to reassure her several times that I did not mind doing the mundane tasks because they are vital to keeping everything flowing as I remember my own TAs carrying out these roles, enabling me to focus on teaching, assessment and planning.

A few times, the children sometimes behaved differently for me when the classteacher left the room, for example, with one child once saying, 'you're just a TA'. He was spoken to by the classteacher, that a TA commands just as much respect as the teacher but that I also was a teacher. I did find the children behaved better for me from then on.

Other members of staff often thought I was training to be a teacher. Having gone from volunteer to TA was a bit confusing for some. In a busy school environment, there isn't always time to speak to everyone individually, so upon reflection I feel the school management should have formally introduced me and my background more to the whole school staff and community in one go. I also went onto see that as other members of staff joined the school after me, I wasn't always sure what their role was: volunteers, students, parent helper, part time etc.

Teaching bubbles during lockdown gave me the confidence to realise that I enjoyed planning and delivering lessons. I then went onto apply for a part-time teaching role at the school.

We can identify that Carrie and the classteacher demonstrate positive attributes of teamwork:

- sharing common goals for the class and their work together;
- providing each other with the support and encouragement to achieve these goals;
- effective communication;
- mutual respect for each other's positions, and this is relayed to other members of the organisation (in this case, the children).

Carrie's reflections continue as she reviews her teaching role during the pandemic.

CASE STUDY 🔂

Carrie, teacher, reflection on transition from teaching assistant to teacher: Part 2

Transitioning to teacher from TA during the pandemic was very tricky. I joined a year group halfway through an already highly disrupted and disjointed year. I found the planning, under Covid-19 restrictions especially, so much more difficult, some of which I have highlighted here.

- *Pressure to know how everything works straightaway as I moved to a different role. As a TA I could easily ask questions for clarification but now as the teacher, I felt responsible for all aspects of the day.*

- *Pressure to follow established systems and planning to support my job share teacher but also to feel like I was pulling my weight with the planning and bringing something new to the role. This was tricky as sometimes the objective from the lead teacher was brief and given at short notice. This was alleviated by learning to assert my boundaries more, making it clear what I needed from the classteacher and by when. I was willing to be very flexible but also couldn't leave things to the last minute. We also started to split the curriculum so I could teach more discrete lessons and not have to worry about continuity so much, with obvious overlap as and when needed, for the children.*

- *I found staff meetings useful to join remotely on my non-teaching days (due to covid restrictions) but this may become an issue going forwards if they are not carried out remotely in the future.*

- *The duration of my teaching days was much longer which I needed to adjust to, regarding my work–life balance.*

- *Quickly it became obvious how crucial the support of a TA is. Some were very supportive and understood it is tricky for a teacher to come into the year group on a part-time basis, part way through the week.*

Critical questions ⑦

» After reading both parts of the case study, what stages from Tuckman's stages of group development can you identify within these two parts?

» Referring to the GRPI model for effective teamwork (Figure 8.1), there are components within this that could be enhanced in Carrie's situation to alleviate her anxieties in the workplace highlighted in part 2. Can you identify these?

» How could you develop the team if you were in a similar position?

Carrie goes on to reflect on some of the power struggles she faced in her role as a part-time teacher in part 3 of her reflection:

CASE STUDY ⊕

Carrie, teacher, reflection on workplace relationship challenges: Part 3

Some support staff were less helpful, not always explaining systems or procedures until it was too late or being unnecessarily attached to their way of doing things, causing me to be sometimes undermined in front of the children.

→

Sometimes I was excluded from conversations about vital assessments and information about individual children when TAs and lunchtime staff communicated only to the main classteacher. I had to again make it clear that it was my job to be aware of what was happening for the well-being of all the children, not simply to assume the role of power or authority. I did feel like some of the TAs who knew the children well didn't seem to respect my authority in the same way as they did with the main classteacher. They would often interrupt during my teaching to reprimand children or become busy with other tasks when they were needed in the classroom. It was tricky finding a balance between giving the TA ownership of tasks but also guiding them to give me the support I needed to achieve the planned objectives. I was sometimes asked to make decisions or provide guidance on matters on the spot, sometimes in the middle of lessons. I had to again assert myself and provide clear boundaries and systems about how I liked to work as otherwise the day would have become overwhelming.

I began to liaise a lot more closely with the classteachers to be aware of issues, problems, safeguarding information etc as much as possible, ahead of time so that I wasn't out of the loop. I took advice from senior management and made sure I planned the tasks and roles I expected the TAs to carry out in order for my lessons to be effective and not for TAs to assume that they could carry on with duties from previously in the week with the other classteacher. I found it difficult to be part of the team, but online tools including Whatsapp and Microsoft Teams helped me to stay connected. In hindsight, I should have appreciated that it would have been tricky for TAs to also adjust to working closely with someone new, and I perhaps could have taken a much more authoritative role in the beginning. I could have requested a meeting with the main classteacher and the TAs together to discuss expectations early on.

Critical questions ⑦

» Can you identify what strategies Carrie adopted to overcome some of the power struggles she faced when working with support staff (TAs and lunchtime staff)?

» Reflect on some of the strategies identified. How could you apply these strategies during your transition into a new role or organisation?

» What power bases (French and Raven, 1959) does Carrie hold as she transitions from TA to teacher role? How could these be used effectively to help her establish her new role as the teacher?

A growth mindset

Negative workplace mindsets can take an insurmountable amount of energy to deal with but even as an individual, you can have the power to make positive changes. Negativity can be contagious and so when someone is constantly complaining or undermining others, it can become self-perpetuating, leading to low staff morale which can also destroy colleagues' trust within a team. This can then affect the productivity of an organisation. Unhappy staff can mean low staff retention, costing the organisation time, money and resources in recruiting new staff (Appelbaum and Roy-Girard, 2007), causing instability, ultimately with the potential to impact on the outcomes for children and families in the care of the organisation. You might now be wondering how you can contribute to a positive workplace. It is important to develop a positive or growth mindset (Dweck, 2006). When starting a new workplace, you need to surround your-self with '*uplifting*' co-workers, stay mentally strong and focus on receiving and giving the best experiences in the organisation (Curnow-Chavex, 2018). It is also important to avoid getting drawn into individual colleague's issues and to challenge negative or fixed mindsets.

Dweck's (2000) '*Self theories*' investigated how people develop beliefs about themselves and how these self-theories create their psychological worlds, shaping thoughts, feelings and behaviours. Through her research on adaptive and maladaptive cognitive-motivational patterns, Dweck's theories reveal why some individuals are motivated to work harder, and why others fall into patterns of helplessness and are self-defeating. We can all attempt to adopt a growth mindset in our lives. For some it requires practice to develop this positive line of thought, for it to become second nature, leaving negative attitudes behind, and for others it may come more naturally. It takes practice and perseverance to maintain a growth mindset.

Self-reflections, solutions and possibilities

As highlighted in Carrie's reflections, it is possible to transition between roles and to estab-lish positive working relationships even when you find yourself in a challenging situation to begin with. It is important to begin a new role or workplace, equipped with knowledge of the organisation, not just the policies and procedures, but of the people that work within it, hence a formal introduction to your new colleagues is essential and a detailed induction pro-cess is required. Understanding the various power bases that individuals hold can also help you to establish clear roles and responsibilities in the workplace.

Moving beyond Tuckman's stages of group development and Beckhard's GRPI model, which identifies the components of effective teamwork, you can establish a positive workplace by adopting some of the methods below.

- **Participative leadership** (Lewin's 1948 and 1997 Democratic leadership style) – using a leadership that involves and engages team members.

- **Effective decision-making** – using a blend of rational and intuitive decision-making methods.

- **Open and clear communication** – ensuring that the team mutually constructs shared meaning and adopts effective communication methods.

- **Valued diversity** – valuing a diversity of experience and background in the team, leading to better decision making and solutions.

- **Mutual trust** – trusting in other team members and trusting in the team as an entity.

- **Managing conflict** – dealing with conflict openly and transparently and not allowing grudges to build up and destroy team morale.

- **Clear goals** – identifying goals and use SMART objectives to develop them; goals must have personal meaning for each team member, building commitment to the organisation.

- **Defined roles and responsibilities** – each team member understands what they must do to support team success.

- **Coordinative relationship** – the bonds between the members allow them to coordinate work to achieve efficiency and effectiveness. Communication is key to this relationship developing.

- **Positive atmosphere** – adopting an overall team culture that is open, transparent, positive, future-focused and able to deliver success.

- **Regular feedback** – seek constructive feedback from colleagues to enhance your teamwork mentality (making it the norm to give and receive feedback) and check that you are still working towards the same organisational goals.

Time to consider ☁

» Using a model of reflection (see Chapter 2), reflect on your own professional practice in terms of your team working skills and ability to transition into a setting or new role.

» How might you enhance or develop your workplace relationships after reviewing this chapter?

Chapter summary 📖

Having considered workplace relationships within this chapter, it appears that communication is key in any organisation. Communication with your colleagues and senior leadership team to ensure that issues are dealt with swiftly and effectively is vital. There is nothing worse than letting an issue fester and potentially defeat an individual into disliking their work. The last thing you want to do is feel like you must resign from a post because of a toxic workplace environment or feel that you are the reason that a colleague is unhappy in their work. Adopting a growth mindset and seeking colleagues who have a similar approach will support a positive workplace environment.

If we can understand how theory underpins our practice, we can begin to apply theoretical knowledge to the motivations of individuals in the organisation, to work more effectively with each other and ultimately progress the profile of an organisation and proficiency for its stakeholders. Applying some of the theories covered in this chapter may support you in your initial steps.

When transitioning into a new role or workplace, it is important to be prepared, to be flexible, to reflect when things are going well and not so well, so that you can develop the strategies to overcome challenging situations with colleagues or to develop the effectiveness of your team. Having a formal induction process with clear expectations for both employee and employer can help mitigate against the 'unknown', ensure clear goals are identified and achieved, boundaries are established and that you are fully prepared to take on your new role.

Further reading

Bradford, H (2012) *The Wellbeing of Children Under Three.* London: Taylor & Francis. Chapter 3: Wellbeing, the early years practitioner and the early years setting.

- This chapter explores the importance of practitioners' individual well-being and considers the impact that this can have on the learning environment.

Curnow-Chavez, A (2018) Four Ways to Deal with a Toxic Co-worker. *Harvard Business Review.* [online] Available at: https://hbr.org/2018/04/4-ways-to-deal-with-a-toxic-coworker (accessed 16 August 2021).

- This article provides a perspective of what a toxic work environment could look like and strategies to handle this in the workplace.

Prowle, A and Hodgkins, A (2020) *Making a Difference with Children and Families: Re-imagining the Role of the Practitioner.* London: Red Globe Press. Chapter 7: The communicating and collaborating practitioner.

- This chapter explores the concept and importance of communication when working with children and families and collaborative working.

Raven, B, H (2004) *Power, Six Bases of Encyclopedia of Leadership.* [online] Available at: https://study.sagepub.com/sites/default/files/reference1.4.pdf (accessed 16 September 2021).

- This publication provides a summary of French and Raven's (1959) different power bases which they identified in their research.

References

Accipio (2021) The GRPI Model. [Online] Available at: www.accipio.com/eleadership/mod/wiki/view.php?id=1928 (accessed 28 October 2021).

Appelbaum, S H and Roy-Girard, D (2007) Toxins in the Workplace: Effect on Organizations and Employees. *Corporate Governance: The International Journal of Business in Society*, 7(1): 17–28.

Beckhard, R (1972) Optimizing Team Building Effort. *Journal of Contemporary Business*, 1(3): 23–32.

Curnow-Chavez, A (2018) *Four Ways to Deal with a Toxic Co-worker.* Harvard Business Review. [online] Available at: https://hbr.org/2018/04/4-ways-to-deal-with-a-toxic-coworker (accessed 16 August 2021).

Dweck, C S (2000) *Self-theories: Their Role in Motivation, Personality, and Development.* Hove: Psychology Press.

Dweck, C S (2006) *Mindset: The New Psychology of Success*. New York: Random House.

Emerson, R M (1962) Power-dependence Relations: Two Experiments. *Sociometry*, 27: 282–98.

French, J R P and Raven, B H (1959) *The Bases of Social Power*. In Cartwright, D (ed) *Studies in Social Power* (pp 150–67). Ann Arbor, MI: Institute for Social Research.

GoodTherapy.org (2019) *Power*. [online] Available at: www.goodtherapy.org/learn-about-therapy/issues/power (accessed 16 August 2021).

Harder, H, G, Wagner, S and Rash, J (2014) *Mental Illness in the Workplace: Psychological Disability Management*. Oxford: Routledge.

Lewin, K (1948) *Resolving Social Conflicts*. New York: Harper & Row.

Lewin, K (1997) *Resolving Social Conflicts & Field Theory in Social Science*. Washington, DC: American Psychological Association.

Manivannan, V (2020) Four Factors that Drive Team Productivity. [online] Available at: https://medium.com/@vardhini.m25/4-factors-that-drive-team-productivity-based-on-the-grpi-model-aadf48d59c (accessed 28 October 2021).

Martinez, A D, Kane, R E, Ferris, G R and Brooks, C D (2012) Power in Leader-Follower Work Relationships. *Journal of Leadership and Organisational Studies*, 19(2): 142–51.

Pfeffer, J (1992) *Managing with Power*. Cambridge, MA: Harvard University Press.

Raue, S, Tang, S, Weiland, C and Wenzlik, C (2013) *White Paper Draft The GRPI Model – An Approach for Team Development*. [online] Available at: https://hsrc.himmelfarb.gwu.edu/cgi/viewcontent.cgi?referer=&httpsredir=1&filename=0&article=1017&context=elearning&type=additional (accessed 16 August 2021).

Raven, B H (2004) *Power, Six Bases of, Encyclopedia of Leadership*. [online] Available at: https://study.sagepub.com/sites/default/files/reference1.4.pdf (accessed 16 August 2021).

Tuckman, B W (1965) Developmental Sequence in Small Groups. *Psychological Bulletin*, 63: 384–99.

Tuckman, B W and Jensen, M A C (1977) Stages of Small-Group Development Revisited. *Group & Organization Studies*, 2(4): 419–27. doi: 10.1177/105960117700200404.

Weber, M (1947) *The Theory of Social and Economic Organization*. Oxford: Oxford University Press.

9 Who are your coaches and mentors?

ROSIE WALKER

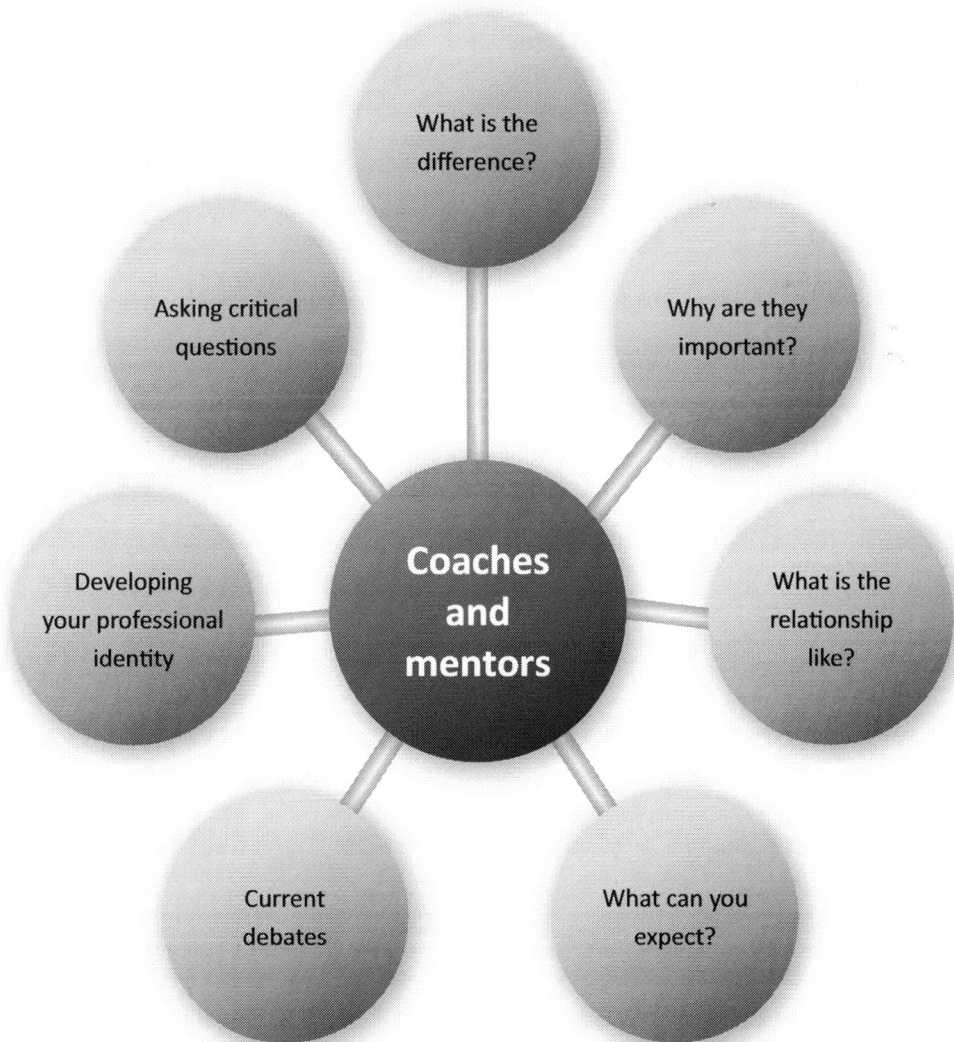

Chapter objectives ◎

This chapter introduces the importance of coaching and mentoring within your career in child and family support. It:

* uses theory and examples to build your understanding of the process of coaching and mentoring and what it has to offer;

* highlights how you can influence and make the best use of what is offered at your setting;

* considers how coaching and mentoring can develop your professional identity and how this might best work for you what can be achieved for your professional development.

When considering coaching and mentoring, introductions are key in cementing a fruitful relationship with your coach or mentor. Building trust at the outset is the foundation of the relationship. So, I would like to introduce myself to you as experiencing both good, bad and indifferent coaching and mentoring, and making use of these experiences when becoming a coach and mentor myself throughout my long career in social care, voluntary organisations and educational settings.

Introduction

Developing professional identity is a key part of offering a quality service to children and families. While this largely comes with experience, coaching and mentoring can be effective in guiding you along the way. Indeed, viewed positively coaching and mentoring can be invaluable in enabling you to nurture your personal and professional growth and development and help you to work effectively with colleagues and children and families to achieve the best outcomes.

Coaching and mentoring within educational, health and social care settings have been expanding in recent years. For example, within early years, it is a statutory requirement in England for all staff to have regular supervision or professional conversations (Department of Education, 2017). Coaching and mentoring play an important part within this remit. It is a requirement because working within these areas can be stressful as there are many demands placed on professionals. Within the early years, for example, there have been changes in legislation and guidance, new demands for safeguarding children, changing curriculums, a call for early intervention and collaborative working as well as responding to inspections and being active in addressing issues of social inequality (Walker, 2021). As Reed and Walker (2017) assert, policies and systems are increasingly defining, refining and shaping children's learning environments. This may be appropriate to the changing world but those working in children and family support need the opportunity to understand, question and challenge these changes. Regular meetings for coaching and mentoring can provide a safe space to facilitate reflective discussion, build on positives, help to assist understanding, and deal with pressures and challenges and look at ways forward (McMahon et al, 2016).

Definitions of coaching and mentoring

Before looking further at how coaching and mentoring might work, these terms need to be defined and the distinctions between them made clear. While they both have factors in common, mentoring usually involves a more experienced, senior person supporting the professional development of the mentee by providing advice and guidance. In contrast, coaching is a more personal approach whereby a goal or vision on which to work is identified. It uses a positive approach to empower development or potential (Reed and Walker, 2020). Starr (2014, p 3) highlights, '*A mentor is someone who takes on the role of a trusted adviser, supporter, teacher and wise counsel to another person*' whereas coaching is defined by Bachkirova et al (2014, p 1) as: '*... a human development process that involves structured, focused interaction and the use of appropriate strategies, tools and techniques to promote desirable and sustainable change for the benefit of the coachee and potentially for other stakeholders*'. Coaching can be defined as a short-term collaborative relationship and perhaps most helpful when you are new to your role, or when new practices are being implemented within the team or workplace. Mentoring is more of an ongoing relationship during transitions in knowledge, thinking or skills to facilitate professional growth (Morgan and Rochford, 2017).

It is useful to decide which of these can best help you within your role and how they can develop your professional identity at any given time. Some settings may not offer a choice and it may be that you can develop a mentoring relationship from another setting. Setting the parameters of a coaching or mentoring relationship is an important part of having a rewarding experience.

It is vital that you recognise who can help you within your role and how you can reach out to them if coaching or mentoring is not readily offered by the setting. This might be, for example, because of the pressure of time to connect with one another to plan or discuss professional issues. This can lead to feelings of isolation, without the benefit of hearing other perspectives and working as a team. Alternatively, some settings may feel that they have little money to invest in coaching and mentoring. This may mean that the service is not offered or is not sustained within some settings, so it is important to establish at interview, start of placement or during induction what is available to you, either as mandatory or good practice. The most effective organisations are those which have a positive and highly motivated culture of coaching and mentoring (Morgan and Rochford, 2017). This is especially important for children and family support work where there are often feelings that the work is undervalued, underfunded and underpaid and a relationship with a mentor can help to sustain staff and reflective listening and questioning can enable workers to realise the importance of the work they are doing (Doan, 2020).

Time to consider 💭

Think about any coaching and mentoring you have already experienced.

» Which coaching or mentoring opportunities have you identified as available to you in your professional role?

> » How successful was it for you and what made it a positive experience? What would you have changed and why? Try to characterise the relationship you had with the coach or mentor and what made it useful?
>
> » What questions would you ask a setting before joining to ensure appropriate coaching or mentoring for you?
>
> » How could you talk to a setting about the need for coaching and mentoring if none is on offer?

What is a coaching and mentoring relationship like?

Having established what coaching and mentoring is, it is useful to have an idea of the relationship you will have with a coach or mentor so you will know what to expect and what to ask for. Of course, each relationship will provide a different experience as we are all human and relate in different ways to one another.

As alluded to in the last section, coaching and mentoring do have common factors and trust between the coach or mentor and coachee and mentee is key to both. This cannot be assumed and must be developed and built on. As Gasper (2020) asserts, this can start to be built by setting the purpose, structure, boundaries and acknowledging that the process is two-way. It can be thought that the mentor or coach has the expertise and is much more knowledgeable than the mentee or coachee. However, this is not always the case and the relationship should be viewed as one where one can learn from the other. A successful mentor or coach will recognise that your work is complex, messy and requires both of you to learn from each other (Pacini-Ketchabaw et al, 2015). Having said that, it is helpful if the coach or mentor understands the organisation in which you work and the requirements of working with children and their families.

Shared ground rules and principles agreed from the start of the relationship and regularly reviewed reinforces mutual respect and an equal partnership. It is important not to slip into a position where the mentee or coachee sees the coach or mentor as 'help', inferring helplessness on their part (Starr, 2014). There can be a delicate balance between what is appropriate to disclose and discuss within sessions and this means that the remit of the sessions needs to be clarified throughout and more complex personal issues may need to be signposted elsewhere. The coaching and mentoring sessions cannot be seen as therapy for personal issues, although the outcome may be therapeutic in moving the coachee or mentee on in their thinking and actions.

These agreements can be seen as a form of contract between the parties, set up at the outset and reviewed at agreed intervals. The organisation may have structures that facilitate this, for example, formal probation paperwork or clinical supervision formats. Ethical practice within the profession can guide and support here. Both parties are encouraged to own the shared process and to recognise confidentiality within the sessions tempered with an understanding of what information may need to be shared elsewhere, for instance in relation to safeguarding or to issues requiring more expert and targeted help.

The issue of power dynamics within the relationship is one that needs to be acknowledged and explored. This is considered further in Chapter 8. While it is the ideal that the relationship is based on mutuality and shared ownership with each learning from the other, there can be situations where the power is not shared equally. For example, the coach or mentor is the leader of the setting and in authority in terms of line management and accountability. Reed and Walker (2020) introduce the notion of horizontal and vertical coaching and mentoring as a way of considering these issues. Horizontal coaching and mentoring entail the mentor or coach imparting information and knowledge with the aim of developing the coachee or mentee's practice and as such can have some benefits. In contrast, a vertical relationship is one where Hammer et al (2014, p 8) suggest *'putting the issue of power on the table'* to develop a *power with* rather than *power over* relationship. In this way discussion can become a valuable learning experience for both parties and is an ethical approach that allows for transparency and safeguards the integrity of the process. An example of a power dynamic might be where a coach or mentor feels it would be appropriate to challenge the coachee or mentee on an issue or a perspective and this is perceived as exerting power over them. A shared discussion and openness can enable deeper understandings to emerge. The preparatory work undertaken in building trust will help to explore uncertainties and more difficult areas. Starting from a position of strengths-based practice building on the positives and the mentee's perspectives, hopes, fears and goals are integral to developing confidence in the relationship.

Listening plays an important part in how trust can be developed. *'Active listening'* (Parsloe and Needham, 2009, pp 141–5) is a key skill for both parties: concentrating on what is being said and teasing out what is not being said. Sensitive, reflective questioning can really open out discussion and allow situations to be considered from different perspectives. This skill is also needed, developed and used in child and family work and will be considered further in the next section.

CASE STUDIES

Examples of horizontal and vertical coaching

Scenario 1

Anna is a new Family Support worker in Primary School Pastoral Support Team. After three weeks of Induction, she is offered the chance to participate in team mentoring attended by her line manager. Within the monthly sessions, the team members take it in turn to bring a concern or an issue to the meeting. An action-based approach is used to enable the team member to firstly outline the issue without interruption. Following this, the team members can ask questions and offer solutions. Information is imparted and actions discussed without the line manager. Each team member takes a turn at leading the mentoring sessions.

Scenario 2

Anna is also provided with mentoring from her line manager initially weekly and then fortnightly. Anna is accountable to her line manager who has authority over her. Together they discuss Anna's workload and individual cases using a strengths-based approach to identify actions and needs within the families and to work on Anna's developing needs as a professional. These sessions are recorded by the line manager and agreed by Anna.

> ### *Time to consider* ☁
>
> » Identify which scenario is vertical coaching and which is horizontal.
>
> » How might vertical and horizontal coaching and mentoring be used in your setting?

What to expect from coaching and mentoring

Having introduced ourselves and set the contract for the chapter, you may by now be getting to know what the chapter is about and feel more at ease with continuing to read it. So too with mentoring and coaching sessions. Once the initial rapport has been made and the contract agreed, it is time to move on to exploring the issues you want to address. It is useful to consider what can be expected so that your needs may be met. If you feel that coaching or mentoring has been imposed upon you, it is likely the sessions will be less successful. Therefore, your attitude before embarking on the process is an important factor. If this is an issue, it needs to be addressed before the process can start so it is important for this to be flagged up early (Harrison, 2020).

The practicalities of what to expect from coaching and mentoring are useful to have in mind when embarking on sessions. Regular meetings set up and planned in advance are helpful in developing a secure basis for the coaching or mentoring. Each meeting should be time limited, with a starting point, a progression, and an end point where the discussion can be summed up and if necessary new goals or areas for discussion can be set.

Location needs to be considered. Should the sessions take place inside or outside the workplace? This depends on the context and whether there is a reliably free space within the setting. The location should be comfortable, with no interruptions so sometimes a busy setting is not a suitable venue. Jewson-Poulter (2020) suggests that the meetings should last for about an hour so that participants do not feel rushed and feel listened to and have time for professional reflection. Having a structure in highly stressful occupations such as social care can provide security and a '*safe space*' to allow the coachee or mentee to step back from the situation and acknowledge and consider their emotional response to allow an objective perspective to emerge (Marjella-Richards, 2020).

The coach or mentor should start from where you are at and listen to your issues. Also, they will make you feel secure to talk about these by setting the ground rules and discussing confidentiality with you. It is useful to have prepared before the meetings to get the best out of them. As mentioned above, there is an expectation that the coach or mentor will be able to listen actively and effectively and to notice body language, nuances of speech and emotion. They will also be able to question by showing curiosity and interest in the dialogue. They will ask open questions to allow expansion of thoughts and will be able to help you to see issues more clearly. For example, if you hold a sheet of paper with writing on it close to your eyes, you will not be able to make out what it is saying. If you hold it further away, you will be able to read it clearly. So, with coaching and mentoring – the coach or mentor will help you to hold issues at arm's length so you can see them clearly and decide how to respond. The listener should also be able to keep track of emerging themes and bring these together for discussion.

It is likely that the coach or mentor will be comfortable with silences and should be able to give space for silence to develop to clarify thoughts. It may well be that this is difficult for the mentee, particularly at first, as many of us rush to fill silence. Try to become comfortable with silence as it can be helpful in providing valuable insights, thinking about a question or its answer or developing a protected space where '*magical understanding unfolds or moments are grasped to clarify both actions and thoughts*' (Turner, 2017, no page number).

It could be said that these skills are part of the coach or mentor's toolbox to enable you to get the best from the sessions. This will also include a non-judgemental approach which can be more evident in mentoring than coaching or supervision where challenges may have to be made. For example, if changes must be made in a setting due to legal requirements and staff are reluctant to change their practice, the coach may need to assert the aims of the organisation. They will be firmer or more directive in their approach while explaining the need for change and understanding the barriers. Both coaches and mentors may need to say difficult things which are hard to hear and saying this in such a way as the participant can hear and recognise the truth of it. However, you should be assured that they will be able to listen to issues that are challenging or disturbing should you need to air these and be able to deal with anger or distress if necessary (Gasper, 2020). Finding the right balance of challenge and support is critical. The coach and mentor should be able to remain calm and always composed and to be professional in their response to you. A coach or mentor should be able to act as a role model for professional practice.

Critical questions ⑦

» What examples can you give of being actively listened to and how that felt?

» How can you develop being comfortable with silence?

Spotlight on new debates

We are living in changing landscapes of practice which have led to more complex ethical and equity dilemmas which require continual criticality and professionalisation in engagement with the issues. This is particularly pertinent in the aftermath of Covid-19 lockdowns and the continuing adjustment to life as a result of the pandemic. In view of this, innovative and creative new ways of communicating and developing coaching and mentoring are needed. For example, due to Covid-19, many people now work from home, and this may mean that supportive conversations no longer take place by the photocopier or the coffee machine. Many people work in isolation or hotdesk. Busy schedules and part-time working may have implications for meetings. New ways of coaching and mentoring such as peer mentoring, emails, online platforms and phone conversations are needed to ensure the safe space practitioners require to engage in professional conversations and explore issues that they encounter.

One way of providing coaching and mentoring differently is to support each other through peer-mentoring. Whether it is through an email, phone call or face-to-face meetings, peer-mentors work together to engage with issues of practice, take a break from the day-to-day work, opting instead to reflect and problem solve through potential issues.

There are several different ways of facilitating peer-mentoring. One example is introduced by Elfer and Wilson (2021, p 6) as a '*work discussion*'. This is where a group of practitioners (5–10 in number) meet regularly for a period of about 60–90 minutes. One member of the group presents their work, aided by the facilitator and the other group members discuss and ask questions to gain new perspectives and develop thinking. Mentoring and coaching, therefore, may need not be a hierarchical relationship where the power and control lie with the mentor or coach: it is possible, for example, for a colleague in a subordinate position to mentor or coach a senior. Where there is a recognition that both are learning from the process and value placed on a culture of respectful relationships, effective coaching and mentoring through this method is likely to flourish.

Whichever method may be decided upon, the leader plays a key role. For example, in times of budget restriction post-covid, it may be difficult and unsustainable to provide every member of staff with coaching or mentoring. A more effective model may be to provide this for the leader who can then support colleagues and staff. This might be offered in several ways, for example, circles of learning or the leader training others to coach or mentor.

Gaining belief in yourself and your practice

Disposition or qualities and general attitude to circumstances as a child, adolescent, student or professional are acquired over time and through a range of your experiences in the life course. These can inform our perceptions of who we are and of our place in the world and the same applies to professional contexts. Some of these issues have been explored in earlier chapters (eg in Chapters 1, 7 and 10). Having safe and sound coaching or mentoring within your supervision is key to your developing professionalism as you progress on the journey of formulating, holding and testing out, re-evaluating and reconstructing your professional values over time.

Shaik and Ebrahim (2020) refer to five states in coaching and mentoring:

1. *Efficacy* relates to an individual knowing that they can make a difference and is willing to do so.

2. *Flexibility* relates to coaching to see a perspective from another angle and not just maintaining one's own view.

3. *Consciousness* is capacity to monitor and reflect on oneself. Conscious individuals are self-directed and are aware of their thoughts, feelings and surroundings. Conscious people progress towards their goals by monitoring their own thoughts and behaviours.

4. *Craftsmanship* focuses more on quality than perfection. Individuals take pride in their work and strive for precision, seek elegance, refinement and specificity similar to that of a performer.

5. The final state of mind is *interdependence* which refers to the ability to learn from others and to contribute to a common good.

By developing these, you will come to know yourself as a practitioner and to have confidence in your practice. This means developing the ability to take responsibility and control over events that affect your practice in a setting.

Critical questions ⑦

» How far do you recognise yourself within the five states? Which state might you wish to develop within your professional identity?

» Thinking about professional role models that you have has what traits can you see in them and how can you use this in your own development?

Chapter summary 📖

Endings of the coaching and mentoring are as important as any other part of the process. Stepping back and sharing the journey you have made with the coach or mentor as well as the specific points covered should enable you to recognise your strengths, how these can be used in the future, as well as having strategies and aims going forward. So too with this chapter, it is important to sum up what we have covered and consider what you might read next.

This chapter has argued that coaching and mentoring are vital ingredients to your practice. However, for this to benefit your professional development to its highest potential it needs to be set up well with your needs at any stage in mind. Organisations that foster a culture of inquiry, promoting learning and critical reflection are likely to be at the forefront of good coaching and mentoring practice (Early Education and Care (CoRe, 2011)).

As I wrote in 2017,

> *Coming to know oneself within and through the changing personal and professional landscapes, having a strong value base and reflecting on the wider issues for practice, lifelong learning and the building of communities of practice are a strong basis for success*
>
> (Walker, 2017, p 499)

Such skills afforded by coaching and mentoring are key in managing adversity, challenges and inequalities which are ever-present in professional life. Ensuring that practitioners have their professional voice heard and have the confidence to become powerful and skilful advocates for children is the cornerstone of successful coaching and mentoring.

Key messages

• Decide your coaching or mentoring needs and to negotiate with the setting how these may be met.

- Agree the purpose and boundaries of the coaching or mentoring sessions for a successful working relationship to develop.

- Prepare for sessions so that the time is spent as profitably as possible.

- Consider the practicalities of the sessions carefully.

- The coach or mentor will have a range of skills to help you express your issues, although learning from the sessions is a two-way process.

- Above all, enjoy your experience!

Further reading

Gasper, M and Walker, R (eds) (2020) *Mentoring and Coaching in Early Childhood.* London: Bloomsbury.

- This book will give you an insight into how coaching and mentoring is carried out internationally. It is divided into chapters that give a theory about coaching and mentoring in different countries and case studies that give you practical examples.

McMahon, C, Dyer, M and Barker, C (2016) Mentoring, Coaching and Supervision. In Trodd, L (ed) *The Early Years Handbook for Students and Practitioners.* London: Routledge.

- This chapter will give you practical insights into coaching and mentoring and how these will support professional development.

References

Atkins, L Bolan, R Chaplin, D Harris, D Harrison, J Henshall, A Munn, H and Whale, L (2017) *Mentoring in Early Years Initial Teachers Training.* A report for the London providers. University of Greenwich.

Bachkirova, T Cox, E and Clutterbuck, D (2014) *The Complete Handbook of Coaching* (2nd ed). London: Sage.

CoRE (2011) Competence Requirements in Early Childhood Education and Care. European Commission, Directorate General for Education and Culture Final Report. University of East London, Cass School of Education and University of Ghent, Department for Social Welfare Studies. September 2011. [online] Available at: https://download.ei-ie.org/Docs/WebDepot/CoReResearchDocuments2011.pdf (accessed 30 August 2021).

Department for Education (2017) *Statutory Framework for the Early Years Foundation Stage: Setting the Standards for Learning, Development and Care for Children from Birth to Five.* [online] Available at: www.foundationyears.org.uk/files/2017/03/EYFS_STATUTORY_FRAMEWORK_2017.pdf (accessed 30 August 2021).

Doan, L K (2020) Finding Community through an Induction Support Pilot Project. In Gasper, M and Walker, R (eds) *Coaching and Mentoring in Early Childhood.* London: Bloomsbury.

Elfer, P and Wilson, D (2021) Talking with Feeling: Using Bion to Theorise 'Work Discussion' as a Model of Professional Reflection with Nursery Practitioners. *Pedagogy, Culture and Society.* [online] Available at: www.tandfonline.com/doi/full/10.1080/14681366.2021.1895290 (accessed 20 January 2022).

Gasper, M (2020) Theory of Mentoring and Coaching in Early Childhood. In Gasper, M and Walker, R (eds) *Coaching and Mentoring in Early Childhood*. London: Bloomsbury.

Hammer, T Trepal, H and Speedlin, S (2014) Five Relational Strategies for Mentoring Female Faculty. *Adultspan*, 13(1): 4–14.

Harrison, J (2020) Mentoring for Success for Early Years Teachers: A Research-based Approach. In Gasper, M and Walker, R (eds) *Coaching and Mentoring in Early Childhood*. London: Bloomsbury.

Marjella-Richards, C (2020) 'Is It Safe?' … Creating Safe Reflective Spaces for Child Protection Practice. In Gasper, M and Walker, R (eds) *Coaching and Mentoring in Early Childhood*. London: Bloomsbury.

McMahon, C, Dyer, M and Barker, C (2016) Mentoring, Coaching and Supervision. In Trodd, L (ed) *The Early Years Handbook for Students and Practitioners*. London: Routledge.

Morgan, M and Rochford, S (2017) *Coaching and Mentoring for Frontline Practitioners*. Dublin: Centre for Effective Services.

Pacini-Ketchabaw, N, Kocher, L E and Sanche, A (2015) *Journeys: Reconceptualizing Early Childhood Practices through Pedagogical Narration*. Toronto, ON: University of Toronto Press.

Parsloe, E and Needham, M (2009) *Coaching and Mentoring: Practical Conversations to Improve Learning* (2nd ed). London: Kogan Page.

Passmore, J, Brown, H and Csigas, Z (2017) *The State of Play in European Coaching and Mentoring*. University of Reading. [online] Available at: https://assets.henley.ac.uk/defaultUploads/The-State-of-Play-in-European-Coaching-Mentoring-Executive-Report-2017.pdf?mtime=20171204192802 (accessed 30 August 2021).

Reed, M and Walker, R (2017) Reflections on Professionalism: Driving Forces that Refine and Shape Professional Practice. *JECER*, 6(2): 177–87.

Reed, M and Walker, R (2020) The Importance and Value of Mentoring and Coaching in the Early Years. In Gasper, M and Walker, R (eds) *Coaching and Mentoring in Early Childhood*. London: Bloomsbury.

Shaik, N and Ebrahim, H (2020) Transforming Pedagogy in Early Childhood Education: A South African Perspective. In Gasper, M and Walker, R (eds) *Coaching and Mentoring in Early Childhood*. London: Bloomsbury.

Starr, J (2014) *The Mentoring Manual: Your Step by Step Guide to Being a Mentor*. Harlow: Pearson.

Turner, A F (2019) *Silence and Its Role in Coaching Practice*. [online] Available at: https://uwe-repository.worktribe.com/OutputFile/1493289 (accessed 30 August 2021).

Walker, R (2017) Learning Is Like a Lava Lamp: The Student Journey to Critical Thinking. *Research in Post-Compulsory Education*. https://doi.org/10.1080/13596748.2017.1381293

Walker, R (2022 in press) Holding and keeping the child safe; In McDowall Clark, R, Solvason, C and Webb, R (eds) *Knowing and Understanding the Early Childhood Practitioner*. London: Routledge.

Part 4　Moving forwards

10 Transition from placement to first role

HAZEL RICHARDS

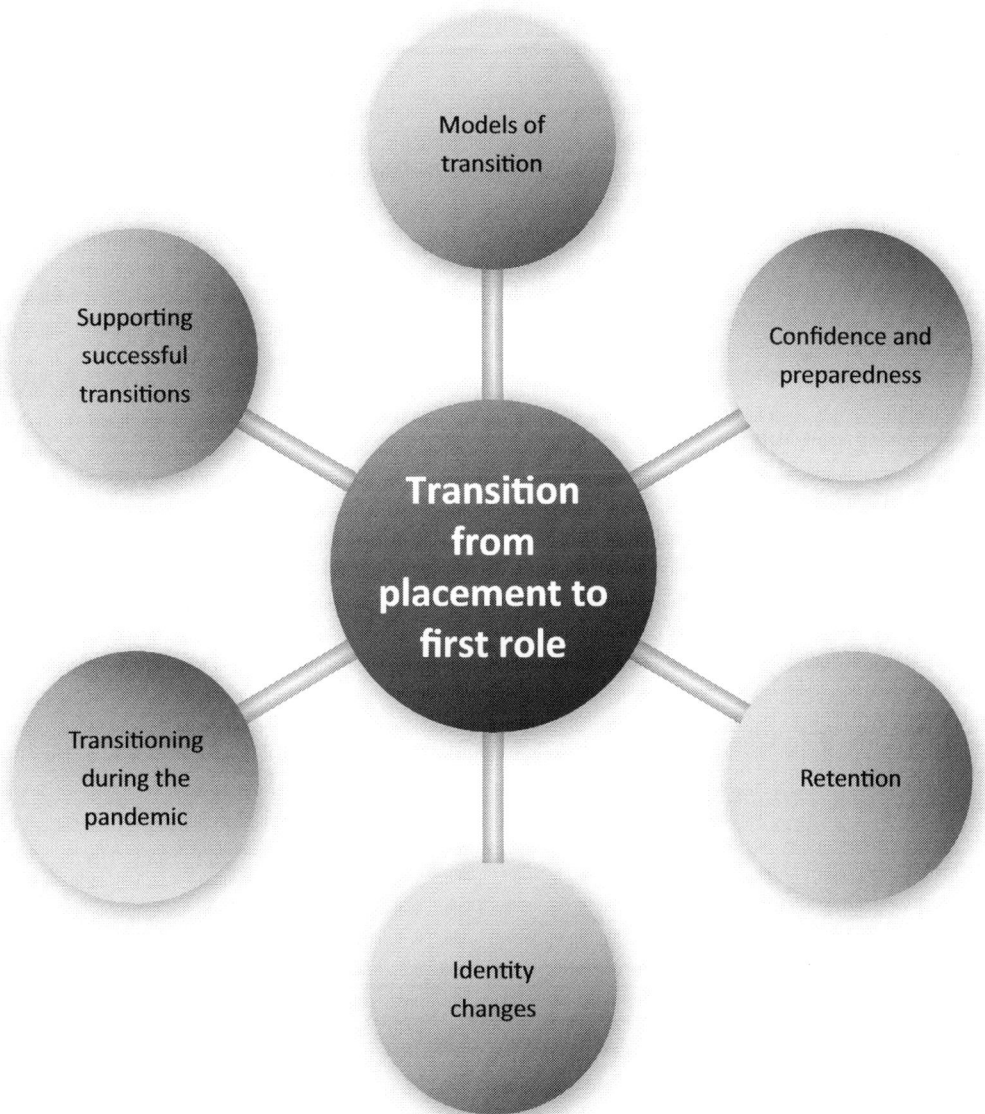

Chapter objectives ◎

This chapter explores transitions from the range of perspectives (education, health and care) involved in child and family support. The chapter:

- introduces you to theories of transition and identity formation;

- poses critical questions to enable you to reflect on your own transition(s);

- considers the unique experience of transitioning from student to the first role during the pandemic;

- suggests how you might support your own transition.

Introduction

Transitions are unique periods in people's lives. Transitioning from student to qualified role and status is a process. Described as a '*rite of passage*' (Bradley, 2008), the first year as a newly qualified practitioner is both important and marked by sudden disruptions and unexpected turns. This is because you do not enter your new role as a completed practitioner. Rather, you will take time to consolidate, clarify and settle into your professional role and identity. Successfully transitioning from being a student to becoming a more proficient practitioner, and adjusting to a new role in an organisation is a process that takes at least 6–12 months (Glasburn, 2018). This is because even though you have learned much about practice on your placements, it is only when you are qualified that you can be exposed to all the realities of the job (Gerrish, 2000). This chapter therefore explores concepts related to transition and identity formation and considers how your own move might be best supported.

Critical questions ⑦

» What differences between your placement and your first role do you anticipate?

» If you have changed role after qualifying, what differences between your old and new role and identity have you noticed?

» How do these differences make you feel?

» What help do you think you need to support your transition? What help is currently in place?

Models of transition

As part of transition, newly qualified practitioners (NQPs) must adapt to new roles, identify and meet changed expectations from colleagues, employers and service-users, and become 'one of the team'. Practitioners moving from practitioner to management roles following their degree must also make these adaptations. Nicholson (1990) suggests four stages are involved in settling into a job role: preparation, encounter, adjustment and stabilisation, whereas Yardley et al (2020), Glaser and Strauss (1971) and Bridges (1986) suggest three key stages:

1.   '*the rite of separation*', which involves endings, anticipating and preparing for responsibility;

2.   '*social limbo*', an in-between stage that involves encounter and adjustment; and

3.   '*reaching a status quo*', which involves stabilisation and becoming part of a team.

In '*the rite of separation*' stage, NQPs must prepare for the change from student to practitioner. This is normally marked by rites of passage such as graduation, which commemorate the end of the formal learning stage and the 'stepping off' or beginning of the next phase. At this stage you will have assimilated a substantial amount of learning and procedural knowledge and will have begun to develop self-knowledge about your individual strengths and weaknesses, approaches to learning, and reflective capacities. This self-knowledge enables you to draw on personal and environmental factors in your new position and to both influence and be influenced by these (Wright, Loughlin and Hall, 2018) and helps you to direct your future learning.

In the '*social limbo*' stage, you may feel you are neither one thing nor another, which can engender feelings of 'otherness'. A '*cloak*' metaphor has been used to denote that although NQPs are able to meet their new responsibilities because of the change in their outward identity conferred by their appointment to the job, most are, in fact, being good actors in that they develop a façade of professionalism, while lacking confidence in themselves (Yardely et al, 2020). The focus of practitioners in this transitional stage is to learn and meet the functional tasks of the job. Engagement in activities that signal compliance with the given professional culture is also important (Hobbs, 2012), so you are unlikely to openly question or suggest changes to practice.

The possibility of being able to participate on both a personal and social level requires NQPs to have a sense of belonging. The process of incorporation (Glaser and Strauss, 1971) and enculturation into a professional community (Lave and Wenger, 1991) involves mutual engagement, joint enterprise and shared repertoires. The final transition stage, '*reaching a status quo*', therefore requires NQPs to '*read*' the workplace culture, become '*system savvy*' (Hobbs, 2012, p 392), and begin to be actively involved with the politics and systems of the practice setting with a view to bringing about change. However, rules of interaction within teams are complex, can be context dependent, and are rarely explicit (Yardely et al, 2020). As an NQP you will therefore be working across personal, professional and collective identities, which will include Imposter Syndrome and thoughts about whether you are 'able' and/or worthy to belong. How strongly you are attached to, and identify with the role, setting and/or organisation will inform your development in this stage, though you may feel conflict and competition as you learn to negotiate the influence and impact of internal and external politics (Wright et al, 2018). Wenger (1998, p 56) therefore suggests that becoming stable requires '*both action and connection; it combines doing, talking, thinking, feeling, and belonging*'. The next section outlines core aspects you may need to consider during your own transition.

Confidence and preparedness

Transitions to practice for newly qualified (NQ) social workers compared to that of other professions, including teachers, nurses and allied health professionals, were explored by Moriarity et al (2011). Graduates across education, health and care reported feeling confident in their knowledge, theory and understanding, but less prepared for managing high caseloads (or managing a workload with limited resources), report writing, record keeping, time management and for specialist practice due to the generalist nature of their education. Moving from the familiar student or previous workplace subculture to the less familiar culture of work can be experienced as a reality or culture shock (Glaser and Strauss, 1971, Yardley et al, 2018) when the lack of congruity between ideal and actual practices (Fenwick et al, 2012) is experienced. This can cause stress, but you may also feel ambivalence about seeking support (Yardley et al, 2018), perceiving that this may reflect negatively on your credibility (Gerrish, 2000) and create extra work for their colleagues. This is important to ponder. Although prior to preceptorship, the mark of a good staff nurse was perceived to be the ability to cope without assistance (ibid), successful transitions are, in fact, enabled by structured support. Gordon (2020) found ongoing linkages (eg with peers), a supportive community of practice, and mentoring were vital, and Kilminster et al (2011) found situational and contextual factors, such as the forming of longitudinal peer-to-peer relationships, contribute significantly to the gaining of confidence and competence.

Independent practice

While a student, independent practice signifies working with little or no assistance under the supervision of a responsible mentor (see Chapter 9). As an NQP, it signifies the ability to practice independently and competently and to become individually and professionally accountable. Independent practice, however, also means recognising when to ask for more help and advice, including when to refer a difficult case for expert input. This means it is also interdependent. Preparedness to acknowledge the limitations of your own expertise and the boundaries or your role is actually a sign of strong responsible practice. Paradoxically, while aspects of independent practice, including decision-making and acting autonomously help us develop responsibility, the identity formation of NQPs is chronologically mismatched with new appointments. Yardely et al (2020) discuss the symbiotic relationship between responsibility and identity as each generate the other through successful actions in practice (Dornan, 2012). While reproduction and maintenance of Professional Standards and practice is important (Hobbs, 2012), independent practice also involves moving beyond replicating our mentors. Adaptation and innovation happen once stabilisation is achieved (Fuchs, 2003). Metamorphosis to independent practice is perhaps therefore achieved when NQPs feel confident to think outside of habitual values (Ingram and Abrahams, 2015), and when they feel able to engage their potential to '*make a difference*' to practice, despite the structural constraints they were required to recognise as part of their transition.

Or not ... retention issues

In contrast to achieving independence, student to professional transitions can involve loss of confidence and periods of struggle (Fenwick et al, 2012). Lack of experience may fuel a lack of confidence, and lack of confidence may fuel uncertainty in the role (Gerrish, 2000). Research shows that NQ teachers struggled to adjust as they moved from the relative safety of the university context to the reality of work 'out' in practice (Gordon, 2020). The challenge of understanding new roles and managing organisational demands certainly cause occupational stress (Allen and Sims, 2018), which has implications for retention. Gordon (2020) found fewer teachers are aspiring to promotion or considering teaching as a lifelong career, and turnover rates within the first five years of qualified practice are 9.2 per cent (teachers, Ward, 2019), 15 per cent (early years, Gov.uk, 2020) and 16 per cent (child and family social workers, DfE, 2019). Glaser and Strauss (1971) contend that the 'reality shock' may be implicated in less-successful transitions. For example, nurses experience degrees of 'thrownness' from challenging situations, which range from being fazed to being the catalyst for rejecting the profession altogether (Hobbs, 2012, p 392). In contrast, in the 'social limbo' stage, increasing competence and familiarity with the work setting can facilitate the confidence required to temper uncertainty. Certainly, Burns, Christie and O'Sullivan (2020) found that if you can retain social workers beyond the five-year point, their retention narrative intensifies, their embeddedness in the organisation and community strengthens and they have a stronger sense of professional confidence as they move out of the early professional stage.

Time to consider 💭

» The section above has explored a range of research from across the sector. As you read this, which points in particular have resonated with you?

» Which aspects have caused you anxiety when transitioning within your professional career?

These aspects are now explored in the following case study.

CASE STUDY ⊙

Laura, 30, lecturer in education

I am the first in my family to ever attend university, and Imposter Syndrome has followed me all my life. I still can't believe that in Spring 2020, I entered my PhD Viva just hoping to pass, with plans to spend the following months on corrections, transitioning out of PhD life. Several hours later I was Dr Laura, no corrections, no transition time, it was over, just like that. I was of course elated, but honestly, panic quickly hit, I wasn't prepared for it to end. As I travelled home nervously refreshing emails for confirmation I wasn't dreaming, I received an interview invitation, and within a week I started my first 'fully-qualified' academic job. Meanwhile, in parallel, Covid-19 had reached the UK and the world turned upside down.

→

I consciously pushed to learn as much as possible throughout my studies and beyond, undertaking research and teaching opportunities, thus experiencing snippets of an academic career. I had a safety net in these roles – as a 'student' nobody would judge requests for guidance, which was great in bolstering me with the confidence to gain experiences that continue to shape my professional identity. But, without that safety net, I falsely thought I was supposed to know everything by the day that I started. I planned to be proactive, based in the office to actively integrate with the department and learn as quickly as possible how to be a 'real' academic. However, this only lasted two weeks as the scale of the pandemic was growing – in a heartbeat, I was working from home, with my Imposter Syndrome for company, trying to adjust to a new job and new responsibilities within a new way of working, to establish what I was doing and hoping it was right.

Now, 18 months later, I continue to navigate how to be doing enough to be worthy of calling myself a lecturer. I love to teach, research, publish, and I even love marking student work, supervising and giving feedback. I still carry my fears, but I'm working on it. I'm just establishing myself in this career, but I have learned throughout this process that even in isolation I am not alone, nor expected to be. Supportive colleagues I have only met through a screen fostered a positive and supportive environment for growth that has made all the difference throughout these transitions. From virtual coffees, feedback and collaborations and making time for what I was worried were the silliest questions, I see that I am part of a collaborative community despite the situational limitations. I have also realised we are all, continually, learning, and that sometimes the best experiences come from sharing our experiences and seeking advice. I am beyond thankful for those who collaborate with me and encourage me as I progress. This, for me, is a journey. I have much to learn, but I'm working on it and have found an amazing community of experience and collaboration that help me get that step closer, every single day.

Time to consider

» What does Laura tell you about her confidence and preparedness?

» Laura states: 'even in isolation I am not alone, nor expected to be' – where or from whom might you receive support from?

» Part of transition involves embedding into the organisation and community. How has Laura managed this, even when working remotely and what might help you do this?

» How successful do you think Laura's transition has been and what are you basing your judgement on?

Identity

Successful transition also involves identity change (Yardley et al, 2020), with the first 12 months identified as an especially important time (Moorhead, 2019) (see Chapter 1). Professional identity is understood as the enactment of core features and norms of a profession, particularly values, ethics and purpose (Wheeler, 2017). The development of these is relational and contextual, so influenced by personal and organisational factors. Educators should therefore consider identity when preparing graduating students for transition to qualified practice. Mentors also need to recognise and support the evolving identity of NQPs.

Core themes related to transition and identity adjustment include using strengths and resilience for positive identity development, drawing on values, applying learning in practice and drawing on relationships. Individuals with strong professional identities demonstrate '*coherence between personal, professional and organisational values*' (Pullen Sansfaçon and Crête, 2016, p 776). Moorhead (2019) identified three questions to be addressed to progress professional identity change.

1. **Consolidating professional identity: who am I as a (*name profession*)?** As an NQP you may be 'thrown in at the deep end'. While this will enable you to gain experience, consolidate your learning and begin to adjust to joining the profession, the resulting growth requires a considerable amount of energy, so there is a need for rest and self-care. As clarity and confidence increase, you will move beyond replication and will start to think about who you want to be as a practitioner, reflecting on your personal style.

2. **Clarifying a distinct professional identity: what are the unique features of (*name profession*) work?** In this stage, you move beyond an individual sense of your specific job to identify features of the profession. Role boundaries become clearer, and you will become more aware of your ethos (eg holistic, child-centred) and be able to identify the value of what you yourself contribute. You will begin to truly identify as a '*name of profession*', though you may still feel that you are 'only just' a *name profession* since you are only just beginning. You are therefore only starting to work out who and what you are in relation to this emergent identity (Wright, Loughlin and Hall, 2018).

3. **Settling into a professional identity: am I worthy and comfortable calling myself a (*name profession*)?** At this stage you will begin to truly identify yourself as a '*name profession*' because you have developed a sense of place within the role. You will have a sense of having earned the right to call yourself a '*name profession*', meaning you feel worthy and comfortable to claim a professional identity as a qualified practitioner, not just an NQP.

Wright et al (2018) observed oscillation along a continuum from master-apprentice, where Newly Qualified Teachers (NQTs) positioned themselves as learning from a more experienced other to a more active engagement with their own professional development. In their pre-service context, NQTs focus on knowledge, teaching skills and competence. Their validation comes from critical engagement and reflection, and from discussions with their peers and educators. However, transition involves leaving that strong, cohesive community of practice (Lave and Wenger, 1991) leading to feelings of uncertainty. Additionally, for those new to the profession and seeking to find not only their place but also their identity, skills and know-how are built up by both successes and failures. Tham and Lynch (2019) investigated social workers' reflections on their first months in practice, finding feelings of unpreparedness, uncertainty about the future and confused perceptions of the workplace. These findings illustrate the vulnerability of NQPs, a finding mirrored in the health literature. What is also mirrored across education, health and care literature is the importance of workplace induction, and the provision of adequate support for NQPs in their new roles.

CASE STUDY ⊕

Sophie, newly qualified children's nurse, general children's ward

I began my role as a staff nurse in September 2020. Working throughout the Covid-19 pandemic gave me little time to think about the transition from student to newly qualified nurse and before I knew it, I was in my blue uniform with sole responsibility for my patients. The fact that my first job was on the same children's ward where I spent many University placements was to my advantage. However, it hit home on my first day that I no longer had the support of a mentor overseeing what I did.

I recall one particularly challenging night shift, where I was the named nurse for five patients, all requiring frequent observations. One patient began to deteriorate at the start of my shift, so I had to prioritise my care around this child. Being newly qualified, I felt nervous about proposing the need for Airvo, as neither the doctors nor experienced nurses had suggested this. However, I knew something needed to be done and eventually it was agreed to place the child on Airvo after which the child's condition improved.

When I finally started to see this improvement, I felt an overwhelming surge of emotions and burst into tears. At this point I was exhausted because I had spent the first half of my shift chasing the doctors and felt I had not done enough. I also had not allowed myself a break or drink until I saw improvement as I was the named nurse responsible for this child's care.

One nurse could see how upset I was and spent time with me to reflect on what had happened, and I realised that if it wasn't for me speaking up and constantly chasing the doctors then this child would have deteriorated further. Although challenging, I believe my confidence in my own abilities grew from this situation, but it has also made me aware of how important it is to speak up when I am worried to ensure the best outcomes for children in my care. It also highlighted the importance of providing myself with a break to prevent burnout during a shift.

Now, in September 2021, I realise just how far I have come despite my transition from student nurse to newly qualified nurse resembling a duck in water – trying to stay above the surface, composed and calm on the outside but underneath the surface, paddling frantically to try and stay afloat. I feared asking questions, as I did not want colleagues to view me as incompetent. However, I realise now that asking for help is not a sign of weakness but a sign of strength – one of the only ways to develop is through utilising the skills and knowledge of others. Although challenging, I feel I have successfully transitioned and am proud of my personal and professional development – so much so that I have recently secured a school nurse position, which I will initially complete alongside my ward-based job. This will allow me to continue to develop my experience, until I feel ready to become a school nurse full-time.

Time to consider 💭

»   Sophie highlights an important dilemma – how to fulfil important responsibilities and still care for the carer. How might she resolve this in future?

»   Can you think of a time when have you have experienced such conflicting demands?

»   Sophie identified the benefit of emotional support and of asking questions. Who are the people you could go to for support and with your questions?

»   How might Sophie's next career transition be different to her first one?

Spotlight on new debates

Covid-19

A transition begins when reality presents an event that changes the patterns of life. This can certainly be said of Covid-19, which required NQPs to cope with new professional work alongside personal challenges. Covid-19 also created a situation during which students considered to be key workers underwent abrupt and early transitions to the professional world (Rodrígues-Monforte et al, 2021). While we cannot fully predict the effects this premature transition has had for these early career practitioners, we can consider elements embedded in this process to gain understanding.

In the initial stages, pre-qualification key workers experienced dangers associated with frontline care due to limited availability of PPE and reduced time for proper supervision and monitoring by qualified and experienced practitioners. Ethical issues were also present. For example: how to allocate limited resources; online practice protocols; balancing the needs of different parties; deciding whether to break or bend policies in the interests of service users; and handling emotions (Banks et al, 2020). As lockdown progressed, the increase in mental health issues (Marsh and Hill, 2020) and safeguarding cases (Gov.uk, 2021) which carries an impact for workers (Nelinger et al, 2021) became apparent.

Transition experiences should enable the development of adaptation and healthy coping strategies, provided circumstances facilitate the process. Normally, transition from student to first qualified role is a predictable, if still somewhat unsettling process, aided by mentoring and support systems. However, the abrupt and premature transition experienced by the graduates of 2020 challenged the process and support mechanisms normally provided (Majrashi et al, 2021). For example: Courtier et al (2021) identified professional socialisation to be a casualty; Rodrígues-Monforte et al (2021) document that nursing student's emotions ranged from excitement to anxiety, sadness, uncertainty and fear; Savitsky et al (2020) found the prevalence of moderate to severe anxiety in nursing students has been 43 per cent and 13 per cent respectively during Covid-19; and McKenzie et al (2021) found the preceptorship programme (NHS Employers, 2021) provided in the first four months following qualification was not carried out during the pandemic.

In contrast to these challenges, Rodrígues-Monforte et al (2021) found students manifested greater professional commitment and a reinforcement of their vocation through this experience, while one of Lightfoot's (2020) teacher participants felt they *'thrive on stressful situations'*. Banks et al (2020) suggest the pandemic highlights many political, professional and personal challenges for policymakers, practitioners and the children and families whom we support. At the heart of these challenges lie ethical questions. Pondering these will contribute to our identity, stance and development as practitioners.

Time to consider 💭

In the pandemic crisis, what helped you to:

» feel welcome and protected in your team?

» provide safe care?

» What were your fears and were they acknowledged?

» If you did enter the workforce prematurely, what impact has it had on your perception of your profession and your future in it?

» What are your suggestions for helping future graduates successfully transition to your team?

What the pandemic and early transition have also highlighted is the reality of emotions and fatigue, and the need for self-care when working in unsafe and stressful circumstances.

Promoting a successful transition

This section explores strategies and support that can promote successful transitions. It is, however, important to bear in mind that transition is a continuum, an ongoing process, marked by lifelong learning and more or less intense periods across the course of a career.

Individually implemented factors

Successful transition involves much more than knowledge and skill acquisition. Transitions offer valuable opportunities for personal and professional development while provoking emotions and requiring energy. 'Becoming' means moving from the safe learning and support zone provided by your tutors and fellow students to take on the mantle of the professional – when you will be viewed by your employer and the children and families with whom you now work as the one who is 'expert' and 'in charge'. This obviously carries attendant expectations and responsibilities (Wright, Loughlin and Hall, 2018), which is both exciting and scary. NQPs are therefore advised to keep a reflexive diary to explore their experiences and encounters in more depth, to identify and develop strategies for the future (Hobbs et al, 2012), and to reflect on their professional identity during the initial post-qualification period (Moorhead, Bell and Bowles, 2016). Exploring and articulating professional identity can make an important contribution to adjustment (Moorhead, 2019). So can building up contacts from within your new team to add to your existing support systems, since fellow team members can relate to the factors present in your specific workplace. Well-being and job satisfaction are influenced by workloads, support and rewards (Ewen et al, 2020), so it is also important that you reflect on these, and that you 'care for the carer' (see Chapter 3). Part of this may be learning to recognise your capacity and saying no. For example, as an NQP you may simultaneously be transitioning into role and expected to support others, for example, students and assistants, a demand that at times may feel like one too many.

Support provided by your context

While higher education institutions need to embed learning in practice and ensure students are provided with authentic and meaningful opportunities (Yardely et al, 2018), they also need to introduce their students to the managerial and organisational skills needed in practice. Similarly, attention should be paid to the bridging period (from the latter part of a degree programme to the end of the first six months in post-qualification post), to address incongruities between students' expectations and the reality in actual settings (Courtier et al, 2021).

NQPs also require structured workplace induction and the provision of adequate support (Tham and Lynch, 2019). This is provided by the 'newly qualified' year (teachers), by the preceptorship programme (nurses), and by the requirement to have competencies signed off (Social Work, Allied Health Professionals and others). However, the quality of transition has been found to be related to how effectively organisations welcomed and supported new graduates in the initial weeks of practice (Phillips, Esterman and Kenny, 2015), with Kilminster et al (2010) finding the practice of NQPs was significantly determined by situational and contextual factors.

Systemic support

Transition mechanisms, in the form of learning and support frameworks, are certainly variably structured in the workplace, but the extent to which NQPs receive support can determine how they gain confidence, autonomy and become part of the team. Internships present an opportunity to develop competencies and put theory into practice so promote professional transitions well (Rodrígues-Monforte et al, 2021). However, the quality of supervision and the adjustment to the professional role, degree of comfort, confidence and competencies of NQPs must also be considered (Kaihlanen et al, 2018). Opportunities for group and peer support, reflection in the form of discussions and debriefing sessions contribute to this, especially since NQPs, may be reluctant to seek help in case this reflects negatively on their credibility. Setting learning objectives during the initial period post-qualification can also be helpful in supporting NQPs through the sometimes challenging process of evolving into resilient and effective children and families support workers.

Chapter summary

Transitioning to your first, qualified role is a staged process. Although mentoring was disrupted by the pandemic, support and strategies can help you successfully progress.

- Personally, you can build your network of support and keep a reflexive diary. This can help you recognise the emotional load of transitioning, chart your changing identity and monitor your well-being.

- Education and work contexts should recognise the importance of the bridging period, including that you may be experiencing incongruities between your expectations and reality. A clear induction and welcoming, supportive atmosphere is important.

- Systematic learning and support mechanisms are also important. This may include progression through a structure with clearly set objectives, and opportunities for peer support and debriefing.

Further reading

Sullivan, S E and Ariss, A A (2021) Making Sense of Different Perspectives on Career Transitions: A Review and Agenda for Future Research. *Human Resource Management Review*, 31(1): 100727 https://doi.org/10.1016/j.hrmr.2019.100727.

- This article covers five theoretical perspectives related to career transition in detail and recognises emerging trends.

References

Allen, R and Sims, S (2018) *The Teacher Gap*. Oxford: Routledge.

Banks, S, Cai, T, de Jonge, E, Shears, J, Shum, M, Sobočan, A M, Stron, K, Truell, R, Úriz, and M J, Weinberg, M (2020) Practicing Ethically during Covid-19: Social Work Challenges and Responses. *International Social Work*, 63(5): 569–83.

Bradley, G (2008) The Induction of Newly Appointed Social Workers: Some Implications for Social Work Educators. *Social Work Education*, 27(4): 349–65.

Bridges, W (1986) Managing Organizational Transitions. *Organizational Dynamics*, 15(1): 24–33.

Burns, K, Christie, A and O'Sullivan, S (2020) Findings from a Longitudinal Qualitative Study of Child Protection Social Workers' Retention: Job Embeddedness, Professional Confidence and Staying Narratives. *British Journal of Social Work*, 50: 1363–81.

Courtier, N, Brown P, Mundy, L, Pope, E, Chivers, E and Williamson, K (2021) Expectations of Therapeutic Radiography Students in Wales about Transitioning to Practice during the Covid-19 Pandemic as Registrants on the HCPC Temporary Register. *Radiography*, 27: 316–21.

DfE (Department for Education) (2019) Experimental Statistics: Children and Family Social Work Workforce in England, Year Ending 30 September 2018. [online] Available at: https://assets.pub lishing.service.gov.uk/government/uploads/system/uploads/attachment_data/file/782154/ Children_s_social_work_workforce_2018_text.pdf (accessed 9 August 2021).

DfE (Department for Education) (2020) Children's Social Work Workforce. [online] Available at: https://explore-education-statistics.service.gov.uk/find-statistics/children-s-social-work-workfo rce#dataDownloads-1 (accessed 9 August 2021).

Donnellan, H and Jack, G (2015) *The Survival Guide for Newly Qualified Child and Family Social Workers: Hitting the Ground Running* (2nd ed). London: Jessica Kingsley Publishers.

Dornan, T (2012) Workplace Learning. *Perspectives in Medical Education*, 1(1): 15–23.

Ewen, C, Jenkins, H, Jackson, C, Jutley-Neilson, J and Galvin, J (2021) Well-being, Job Satisfaction, Stress and Burnout in Speech-Language Pathologists: A Review. *International Journal of Speech-Language Pathology*, 23(2): 180–90.

Fenwick, J, Hammond, A, Raymond, J, Smith, R, Gray, J, Foureur, M, Homer, C and Symon, A (2012) Surviving, not Thriving: A Qualitative Study of Newly Qualified Midwives' Experience of Their Transition to Practice. *Journal of Clinical Nursing*, 21: 2054–63.

Foster, D, Long, R and Danechi, S (2021) *Teacher Recruitment and Retention in England*. Briefing paper number 7222. London: House of Commons Library. [online] Available at: https://commons library.parliament.uk/research-briefings/cbp-7222/ (accessed 3 August 2021).

Fuchs, C (2003) Some Implications of Pierre Bourdieu's Works for a Theory of Social Self Organization. *European Journal of Social Theory*, 6(4): 387–408.

Gerrish, K (2000) Still Fumbling Along? A Comparative Study of the Newly Qualified Nurse's Perception of the Transition from Student to Qualified Nurse. *Journal of Advanced Nursing*, 32(2): 473–80.

Glaser, B G and Strauss, A L (1971) *Status Passage*. London: Routledge and Kegan Paul.

Glassburn, L S (2018) Where's the Roadmap? The Transition from Student to Professional for New Master of Social Work graduates. *Qualitative Social Work*, 19(1): 142–58.

Gordon, A L (2020) Educate – Mentor – Nurture: Improving the Transition from Initial Teacher Education to Qualified Teacher Status and Beyond. *Journal of Education for Teaching*, 46(5): 664–75.

Gov.uk (2020) Stability of the Early Years Workforce in England Report. [online] Available at: www. gov.uk/government/news/stability-of-the-early-years-workforce-in-england-report (accessed 9 August 2021).

Harrison, G and Healy, K (2015) Forging an Identity as a Newly Qualified Worker in the Non-government Community Services Sector. *Australian Social Work*, 69(1): 80–91.

Hobbs, J A (2012) Newly Qualified Midwives' Transition to Qualified Status and Role: Assimilating the 'Habitus' or Reshaping It? *Midwifery*, 28: 391–9.

Ingram, N and Abrahams, J (2015) Stepping Out of Oneself: How a Cleft-Habitus Can Lead to Greater Reflexivity through Occupying 'the Third Space'. In Thatcher, J, Ingram, N, Burke, C and Abrahams, J (eds) *Bourdieu: The Next Generation.* London: Routledge.

Kaihlanen, A M, Haavisto, E, Strandell-Laine, C and Salminen, L (2018) Facilitating the Transition from a Nursing Student to a Registered Nurse in the Final Clinical Practicum: A Scoping Literature Review. *Scandinavian Journal of Caring Sciences,* 32(2): 466–77.

Kilminster, S, Zukas, M, Quinton N, Roberts, T (2011) Preparedness Is not Enough: Understanding Transitions as Critically Intensive Learning Periods. *Medical Education,* 45(10): 1006–15.

Lave, J and Wenger, E (1991) Legitimate Peripheral Participation in Communities of Practice. *In* Harrison, R, Reeve, F, Hanson, A and Clarke, J (eds) *Supporting Lifelong Learning Vol 1: Perspectives on Earning* (pp 111–26). London: Routledge Falmer.

Lefroy, J, Yardley, S, Kinston, R, Gay, S, McBain, S and McKinley, R (2017) Qualitative Research Using Realist Evaluation to Explain Preparedness for Doctor's Memorable 'Firsts'. *Medical Education,* 51(10): 1037–48.

Lightfoot, L (2020) 'It's been Hard, I'm not Going to Lie': New Teachers First Term in a Covid Pandemic. *The Guardian,* 19 December. [online] Available at: www.theguardian.com/education/2020/dec/19/new-teachers-first-term-in-covid-pandemic (accessed 4 August 2021).

Local Government Association (2021) COVID-19 Adult Safeguarding Insight Project – Second Report (July). [online] Available at: www.local.gov.uk/publications/covid-19-adult-safeguarding-insight-project-second-report-july-2021 (accessed 9 August 2021).

Majrashi, A, Khalil, A, Nagshabandi, E A and Majrashi, A (2021) Stressors and Coping Strategies among Nursing Students during the Covid-19 Pandemic: Scoping Review. *Nursing Reports,* 11(2): 444–59.

Marsh, S and Hill, A (2020) Figures Lay Bare Toll of Pandemic on UK Children's Mental Health. *The Guardian,* 21 October. [online] Available at: www.theguardian.com/society/2020/oct/21/figures-lay-bare-toll-of-pandemic-on-uk-childrens-mental-health (accessed 4 August 2021).

McKenzie, R, Miller, S, Cope, V and Brand, G (2021) Transition Experiences of Newly Qualified Registered Graduate Nurses Employed in a Neonatal Intensive Care Unit. *Intensive and Critical Care Nursing.* doi.org/10.1016/j.iccn2021.103112.

Moorhead, B (2019) Transition and Adjustment to Professional Identity as a Newly Qualified Social Worker. *Australian Social Work,* 72(2): 206–18.

Moorhead, B, Bell, K and Bowles, W (2016) Exploring the Development of Professional Identity with Newly Qualified Social Workers. *Australian Social Work,* 69(4): 456–67.

Moriarity, J, Manthorpe, J, Stevens, M and Hussein, S (2011) Making the Transition: Comparing Research on Newly Qualified Social Workers with Other Professions. *British Journal of Social Work,* 41(7): 1340–56.

Nelinger, A, Album, J, Haynes, A and Rosan, C (2021) *Their Challenges Are Our Challenges.* Anna Freud National Centre for Children and Families. [online] Available at: www.annafreud.org (accessed 27 July 2021).

NHS Employers (2021) *Preceptorships for Newly Qualified Staff.* [online] Available at: www.nhsemployers.org/articles/preceptorships-newly-qualified-staff (accessed 10 August 2021).

Nicholson, N (1990) The Transition Cycle: Causes, Outcomes, Processes and Forms. In Fisher, S and Cooper, C L (eds) *On the Move; The Psychology of Change and Transition.* Chichester: John Wiley.

Phillips, C, Esterman, A, Kenny, A (2015) The Theory of Organisational Socialisation and Its Potential for Improving Transition Experiences for New Graduate Nurses. *Nurse Education Today*, 35: 118–24.

Pullen Sansfaçon, A and Crête, J (2016) Identity Development among Social Workers, from Training to Practice: Results from a Three-Year Qualitative Longitudinal Study. *Social Work Education*, 35(7): 767–79.

Rodrígues-Monforte, M, Berlanga-Fernández, S, Martín-Arribas, A, Carrillo-Álvarez, E, Navarro-Martínez, R and Rifà-Ros, R (2021) Premature Transition of Nursing Students to the Professional World due to COVID-19 Pandemic. Nurse Education in Practice 102997 https://doi.org/10.1016/j.nepr.2021.102997

Savitsky, B, Findling, Y, Ereli, A and Hendel, T (2020) Anxiety and Coping Strategies among Nursing Students during the Covid-19 Pandemic. *Nurse Education in Practice*, 46, 102809.

Tham, P and Lynch, D (2019) 'Lost in Transition?' – Newly Educated Social Workers' Reflections on Their First Months in Practice. *European Journal of Social Work*, 22(3): 400–11.

Ward, H (2019) One in Three Teachers Leaves within Five Years. *Times Education Supplement*, 27 June. [online] Available at: www.tes.com/news/one-three-teachers-leaves-within-five-years (accessed 9 August 2021).

Wenger, E (1998) *Communities of Practice. Learning, Meaning and Identity*. New York: Cambridge University Press.

Wheeler, J (2017) Shaping Identity? The Professional Socialisation of Social Work Students. In Webb, S (ed) *Professional Identity in Social Work* (pp 183–96). New York: Routledge.

Wright, V, Loughlin, T and Hall, V (2018) Exploring Transitions in Notions of Identity as Perceived by Beginning Post-compulsory Teachers. *Research in Post-Compulsory Education*, 23(1): 4–22.

Yardley, S, Kinston, R, Lefroy, J, Gay, S and McKinley, R K (2020) 'What Do We *Do*, Doctor?' Transitions of Identity and Responsibility: A Narrative Analysis. *Advances in Health Sciences Education*, 25: 825–43.

Yardley, S, Westerman, M, Bartlett, M, Walton j M, Smith, J, Pelle, E (2018) The Do's, Don't and Don't Knows of Supporting Transition to more Independent Practice. *Perspectives on Medical Education*, 7: 8–22.

Conclusion

Throughout this book, we have covered key issues that contribute to your developing professional identity so as to support you as you transition into independent, qualified practice. The chapters have included critical questions, time to consider moments and case studies. The critical questions and time to consider moments are intended to help you apply the content to your own situation. Indeed, the case studies give a face and humanness to the chapter contents so function to bridge between theory and how this may be experienced or applied in practice. This means parts of the book have the potential to be emotive.

The introduction outlined our intention for a book which plugs a gap in supporting students and newly qualified practitioners as they join the workforce. Having undergone this shift ourselves, albeit some time ago, and supported many such transitions during our own professional practice, we have more recently witnessed and come to appreciate the identity changes, challenges and uncertainties involved for our students involved in this phase of their career. This book is therefore the product of our desires to achieve support and create a resource for our students in collaboration with others who are experts in relevant fields and who share this passion to support practitioners to develop both capabilities and well-being. It has therefore become, as Wenger (1998) describes, a community of practice.

Each author has been generous in sharing their experiences, insights and knowledge – all gleaned through time spent in the children and families' sector. These are shared to support you as you weave your own professional identity, to enable and empower you while in placement and when establishing yourself within the workforce. Alongside this we acknowledge the power of the case studies within the book, all of which are real experiences of practice. Certainly as editors, we are grateful to each and every contributor and know that by working together we have produced a book that is powerful and practical and which we hope will become a text to go-to as you enter and progress in the sector.

In reflecting on the process of writing and on the content of the book, we recognise that we too have learnt much about ourselves: from our research, from our co-authors and from the case study voices. From Part 1 (Recognising the power of work-based learning), we learned the power of knowledge and relationships (Chapter 1, Developing your identity, agency and voice) and the importance of reflecting on your own identity, attributes, values and beliefs in combination with your practice (Chapter 2, Empowering reflective practice). Part 2 (Caring for yourself as a work-based learner) resulted in pivotal changes in our own self-care. For example, by accessing and applying the resources suggested in the self-care chapter (Chapter 3) we have both identified and begun to implement self-care strategies, whereas the detail in the resilience chapter (Chapter 4) and the empathy, compassion and emotions chapter (Chapter 5) reiterated to us the need to develop an understanding of self – our strengths, triggers and limits as human beings and the need to identify compassionate boundaries.

Moving forward, Part 3 (Succeeding amid work-based learning issues) addresses some of the realities inherent in practice and that you will need to navigate as part of your early experiences and responsibilities. Chapter 6 (Finding your place in safeguarding practice) contains a very relatable account of a practitioner reflecting on finding themselves within this area of practice. Sadly, while writing this conclusion another Serious Case Review has begun, which again highlights the need to open discussions as highlighted in this chapter. Chapter 7 (Understanding and responding to adverse childhood experiences in practice) highlights the voices at the heart of practice within the sector and emphasised to us again the power children's voices have in helping us understand their holistic needs. Chapter 8 (Developing workplace relationships) drew attention to issues we have both experienced and navigated through. Finally, Chapter 9 (Who are your coaches and mentors?) underscored the import-ance, again, of relationships and Chapter 10 (Transition from placement to first role) let us uncover theory, and so understand the stages we ourselves have passed through several times over the course of our careers. Certainly, creating and reading through each chapter has enhanced our own perceptions and knowledge though it is important for you to identify what you have learned and will change as a result of reading this book.

At the very start of this book, we knew we wanted to support the independence and resili-ence of those working in child and family support work. Viewing well-being as a source of capital, the book has sought to support and progress personal development by providing a range of strategies and by signposting resources for you to choose from. It does this in recognition that identity development is not linear, is an ever-evolving process, is unique to each one of us, and in recognition that your needs may change over time and in relation to your circumstances. Indeed, we must avoid complacency and recognise none of us ever have it all completely sussed. We must also recognise that, in line with the focus on iden-tity, that as a human there will be areas of work where your practice may be buoyant and other areas, for example new environments, where it is perhaps less so. Questions about how we do support independence and resilience and how can we support this within the sector therefore remain. The book has identified the need to respect self-care and how this might be addressed systematically within the sector. Indeed, Chapter 3 highlighted a strong connection between self-care, good mental health and well-being including the need to build in space to just be. However, we know disparity in how this is embedded in practice persists.

If we have one hope for this book, it is that self-care is highlighted and normalised and that this book empowers people to be brave, courageous and to question the consistency and commitment to approaches to self-care to ensure it becomes very much part of your professional identity. However, we are aware that despite challenges created by the pandemic increasing the need for self-care, some of these same challenges have diminished opportunities for self-care, for example capacity to support regular coaching and mentoring. We want to challenge this situation and hope that the content of the book creates material that can facilitate solution-focused discussions and responses around this and to be part of the solution to the risk of burnout that many practitioners may experience at one stage or another.

We also know that this book could not have been written without our cohorts of students. In the past 18 months these students have identified issues that have been addressed in the book since working within the sector during a pandemic created new and unique experiences within practice. This has enriched the content and must be attributed to them. Indeed, it is particularly important to understand, in line with Roldan (1992, p 62) that 'experiences, languages and culture (are) strengths to be respected and woven into the fabric of knowledge production and dissemination, not ... deficits that must be devalued, silenced and overrun'. It was therefore always our intention to avoid a prescriptive approach to developing your professional identity.

This is because each of you bring a set of history, experiences and knowledge, unique to you and these will inform the content and solutions that you identify as personally meaningful to you. The book should therefore be used to identify and respond to your own support needs, and you should select the tools and strategies you need at any given time. Certainly, developing a professional identity is an evolving process that is influenced by time, situations, settings, life stages and experiences. In summary we hope that this book supports a strength-based approach to developing your professional identity. Our hope is that the content supports your progression, development, resilience and retention within the sector.

We want to end by expressing how much we value and respect each and every one of you – the practitioners of the future.

Hazel and Michelle

References 📚

Roldàn, L I (1992) From the Barrio to the Academy: Revelations of a Mexican American 'Scholarship Girl'. *New Directions for Community Colleges*, 80: 55–64. [online] Available at: https://laurare ndonnet.files.wordpress.com/2018/07/from-barrio.pdf (accessed 1 December 2021).

Wenger, E (1998) *Communities of Practice: Learning, Meaning, and Identity.* New York: Cambridge University Press.

Index